*Recent Advances in*

# Histopathology
# 20

# Recent Advances in Histopathology 19
*Edited by DG Lowe & JCE Underwood*

ISBN 0-443-063478

ISSN 0-0143 6953

*Recent Advances in*

# Histopathology
# 20

*Edited by*

## David G. Lowe MD FRCS FRCPath FIBiol

Professor of Surgical Pathology, St Bartholomew's and The Royal London
School of Medicine and Dentistry, Queen Mary and Westfield College,
University of London, London, UK

## James C. E. Underwood MD FRCPath

Joseph Hunter Professor of Pathology and Head of Department,
Department of Pathology, University of Sheffield,
Sheffield, UK

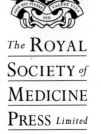

*The* ROYAL
SOCIETY *of*
MEDICINE
PRESS Limited

© 2003 Royal Society of Medicine Press Ltd

1 Wimpole Street, London W1G 0AE, UK

*Customers in North America should order via:*
RSM Press, c/o Jamco Distribution Inc., 1401 Lakeway Drive, Lewisville,
TX 75057, USA. Tel: +1 800 538 1287 (toll free); Fax: +1 972 353 1303.
Email: jamco@majors.com

http://www.rsmpress.co.uk/agents.htm

British Library Cataloguing in Publication Data
A catalogue record for this book is available from the British Library

ISBN 1-85315-511-X

ISSN 0143 6953

Commissioning editor - Peter Richardson
Editorial assistant - Gabrielle Lowis
Production by GM & BA Haddock, Midlothian, UK
Printed in Spain by T.G. Hostench S.A.

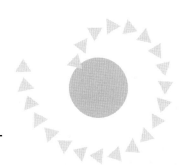

# Contents

# Contributors

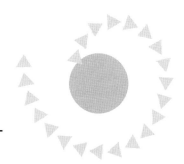

**R.L. Attanoos** BSc MBBS FRCPath
Consultant Pathologist, Department of Histopathology, Llandough Hospital, Cardiff and Vale NHS Trust, Penarth, South Glamorgan, UK

**Clair du Boulay** MSc(Med Ed) DM FRCPath
Director of Medical Education, Southampton University Hospitals NHS Trust, Tremona Road, Southampton, UK

**Andrea Buda** MD PhD
Post-doctoral Clinical Research Fellow, Department of Pathology and Microbiology, Division of Histopathology, University of Bristol, Bristol Royal Infirmary, Bristol, UK

**David Clark** MD MRCP FRCPath
Consultant Histopathologist, United Lincolnshire Hospitals NHS Trust; Honorary Consultant Histopathologist, University Hospital, Nottingham; and Special Lecturer in Pathology, University of Nottingham, Nottingham, UK

**M.S. Fernando** MBBS Dip Pathol, MD (Histopath)
Academic Commonwealth Scholar, Academic Unit of Pathology, University of Sheffield, Medical School, Sheffield, UK

**Peter N. Furness** BM BCh PhD FRCPath
Professor of Renal Pathology, University of Leicester, and Honorary Consultant Histopathologist, University Hospitals of Leicester NHS Trust, Leicester, UK

**A.R. Gibbs** TD MB ChB FRCPath
Consultant Pathologist, Department of Histopathology, Llandough Hospital, Cardiff and Vale NHS Trust, Penarth, South Glamorgan, UK

**Mark K. Heatley** MD FRCPath
Consultant Gynaecological Histopathologist, Department of Histopathology, St James's University Hospital, The Leeds Teaching Hospitals NHS Trust, Leeds, UK

**Kenneth J. Hillan** MBChB FRCS FRCPath
Vice President, Department of Pathology, Genentech, Inc., South San
Francisco, California, USA

**P.G. Ince** BSc MBBS MD FRCPath
Professor of Neuropathology, Academic Unit of Pathology, University of
Sheffield, Medical School, Sheffield, UK

**David G. Lowe** MD FRCS FRCPath FIBiol
Professor of Pathology, Histopathology Department, St Bartholomew's and
Royal London Hospital School of Medicine and Dentistry, Queen Mary and
Westfield College, University of London, London, UK

**Glenn McCluggage** FRCPath
Consultant Pathologist, Department of Pathology, Royal Group of Hospitals
Trust, Belfast, UK

**Anne Marie McNicol** BSc MD MRCP(UK) FRCPGlas FRCPath
Reader in Pathology, Department of Pathology, Glasgow Royal Infirmary,
North Glasgow University Hospitals NHS Trust, Glasgow, UK

**Esther J. Millward** BSc MBChB
SpR Histopathology, Department of Histopathology, St James's University
Hospital, The Leeds Teaching Hospitals NHS Trust, Leeds, UK

**Nina Frances Ockendon** BSc(Hons)
Research Fellow, Department of Pathology and Microbiology, Division of
Histopathology, University of Bristol, Bristol Royal Infirmary, Bristol, UK

**Franklin V. Peale Jr** MD PhD
Associate Director, Department of Pathology, Genentech, Inc., South San
Francisco, California, USA

**Massimo Pignatelli** MD PhD FRCPath
Professor of Histopathology, Department of Pathology and Microbiology,
Division of Histopathology, University of Bristol, Bristol Royal Infirmary,
Bristol, UK

**David Neil Slater** MBChB BMSci FRCPath
Consultant Dermatopathologist, Royal Hallamshire Hospital, Sheffield, UK

**James C.E. Underwood** MD FRCPath
Joseph Hunter Professor of Pathology and Head of Department, Department
of Pathology, University of Sheffield, Sheffield, UK

**S.B. Wharton** BSc MBBS MSc MRCPath
Senior Clinical Lecturer in Neuropathology, Academic Unit of Pathology,
University of Sheffield, Medical School, Sheffield, UK

**Bridget S. Wilkins** DM PhD FRCPath
Consultant Histopathologist, Newcastle upon Tyne Hospitals NHS Trust and
Honorary Senior Lecturer, University of Newcastle upon Tyne, Newcastle
upon Tyne, UK

*Anne Marie McNicol*

**1**

# Criteria for diagnosis of follicular thyroid neoplasms and related conditions

A number of thyroid lesions are characterised by follicular architecture. Most are non-neoplastic or benign, such as dominant nodules in multinodular goitre and follicular adenomas. Follicular variant of papillary carcinoma (FVPC) and follicular carcinoma are the most common of the malignant lesions. Hürthle cell lesions are grouped with follicular tumours in this discussion, as the diagnostic criteria used to assess the behaviour of the two groups are similar. The histological changes caused by fine needle aspiration (FNA) are also discussed, as they may be relevant in the assessment of malignancy. Hyalinising trabecular tumour, follicular variant of medullary carcinoma and mixed follicular and medullary carcinoma are rare differential diagnoses to be considered. This chapter discusses the contributions of cytology, histology and ancillary techniques to the eventual diagnosis and management of the patient.

## CLINICAL PERSPECTIVE

Palpable thyroid nodules are found in 4–7% of the population, and are more common in women and with increasing age. Although the patient or the clinician may have noticed an apparently solitary nodule, the majority are dominant nodules in nodular goitres. Most of the remainder are follicular adenomas. Small non-palpable nodules are increasingly identified when the neck is scanned. The approach to these is still a matter of debate and they are not discussed further here. Thyroid cancer accounts for only 4–10% of palpable nodules, and for about 1.3% of all malignancies and 0.4% of deaths from cancer in the US. An incidence of 0.5–10 cases per 100,000 population has been reported in various geographical regions with 2.3 per 100,000 women and 0.9 per 100,000 men in the UK, where approximately 1000 new cases are recorded each year. The published data would suggest that in areas with adequate

**Dr Anne Marie McNicol** BSc MD MRCP(UK) FRCPGlas FRCPath
Reader in Pathology, Department of Pathology, Glasgow Royal Infirmary, North Glasgow University
Hospitals NHS Trust, Castle Street, Glasgow G4 0SF, UK

iodine intake, about 80% are papillary carcinoma, 10–15% follicular carcinoma and about 10% medullary carcinoma. In iodine-deficient areas, follicular carcinoma is more common and may account for up to 45% of cases. The overall 10-year survival rate for middle-aged adults is 80–90%. However, 5–20% of patients have local or regional recurrence and 10–15% distant metastases: 9% of patients die of their disease with about 275 deaths recorded annually in UK.

Clinical features are of importance in assessing the risk of malignancy. The finding of hard or fixed nodules raises the suspicion of carcinoma, while soft or fluctuant nodules are more usually non-neoplastic or benign. Most carcinomas are 'cold' nodules – that is, they do not show significant uptake of radio-iodine. However, benign thyroid nodules may also show this pattern. 'Hot' nodules that show significant uptake are less likely to be malignant. Four main variables have been shown to have independent poor prognostic relevance in carcinomas: (i) extremes of age; (ii) male gender; (iii) histological evidence of poor differentiation; and (iv) tumour stage.[1] Treatment may also influence prognosis.

Patients with thyroid nodules should be investigated and treated by a multidisciplinary team that includes a pathologist. The aim is to make the correct diagnosis as soon as possible after presentation, to prevent unnecessary surgery and to guide treatment when malignancy is diagnosed. The first approach to a thyroid lump should now be fine needle aspiration (FNA) cytology. This has reduced the number of patients requiring surgery, because a clear diagnosis of benign disease indicates that the nodule need not be removed other than for local pressure effects or cosmetic reasons. This has reduced the need for operative surgery for thyroid nodules by 50%, but has increased the yield of cancers from 10–15% to 20–50%.[2] However, FNA is not yet the norm, and the proportion of patients having FNA varies with the centre. Recent studies from the US and UK suggest that FNA is used as the initial procedure in only 52–84% of patients with thyroid nodules.[3,4]

## FINE NEEDLE ASPIRATION CYTOLOGY

The rule of thumb is that FNA should be performed on a solitary or dominant nodule more than 10 mm in diameter. When the nodule is palpable, it can be aspirated under direct palpation in the first instance. Ultrasound guidance is used for all lesions in some centres. However, in view of the additional resource required, many centres would reserve its use for cases where standard FNA yields non-diagnostic material. It is also especially useful in complex cysts, in lesions that are difficult to palpate and in targeting the dominant nodule(s) in multinodular goitre. Aspiration should be carried out by a clinician with an interest in thyroid disease who is trained in good practice and performs aspirates regularly. This can be a cytopathologist, surgeon, endocrinologist or radiologist. The cytopathologist reporting the FNA should also have an interest in thyroid disease and report sufficient cases to maintain expertise. There should be the opportunity for cytology review, and correlation with any subsequent histology is essential as part of audit. In most centres, a combination of wet and air-dried preparations is used. Additional material may be processed as cytospin slides, cell blocks or Millipore filter preparations for immunohistochemistry where appropriate, or processed for molecular genetic analysis. In most instances, the diagnosis of follicular lesions is made on standard smears.

Aspirates are usually divided into five categories: (i) non-diagnostic; (ii) non-neoplastic and benign; (iii) follicular lesions (usually neoplasms); (iv) suspicious of malignancy (papillary, medullary or anaplastic carcinoma, or lymphoma); and (v) diagnostic of malignancy (in the same range of tumours). A typing system of Thy1–Thy5 has recently been proposed. Published figures suggest that inadequate/non-diagnostic (Thy1) FNAs should be about 5–15% of the total, the figure being lower in ultrasound guided lesions. Specimens are usually considered adequate when they contain at least six groups of 10–20 cells each on two different slides.[5] This baseline is especially important when making a benign diagnosis. A diagnosis of malignancy may be made with fewer cells where the characteristic features are pronounced (*e.g.* papillary carcinoma). Aspirates that cannot be interpreted because of technical artefact also come into the Thy1 category. The discussion that follows highlights the FNA appearances of the range of follicular lesions of the gland. It does not address inflammatory conditions or tumours with a non-follicular architecture.

The aspirate from nodular goitre shows abundant thin colloid, sometimes with a 'cracking' artefact. The follicular cells lie in sheets, follicles or singly. Foamy and haemosiderin-laden macrophages are usually present though their numbers will vary with the extent of degeneration. This will be classified as Thy2. In some cases of hyperplastic nodules, the appearances will fall within the spectrum more usually associated with follicular neoplasms (Thy3). Some would advocate that a benign diagnosis should be made confidently only on the basis of two aspirates, 3–6 months apart. However, others would not recommend a repeat if the first aspirate is adequate and the nodule is < 20 mm in diameter and not increasing in size.

The third category (Thy3) comprises mainly follicular neoplasms. Follicular Hürthle cell tumours are included in this group. It is not possible to make the distinction between benign and malignant tumours on cytology alone, and all cases in this group require lobectomy for definitive diagnosis. The majority of these lesions are follicular adenomas, with up to 15% reported as follicular carcinomas. These are cellular aspirates, comprising follicular or Hürthle cells arranged in microfollicles or three-dimensional groups, with little colloid. Nuclear atypia may be seen, but is not important in defining the behaviour of the lesion as atypical adenoma may show pleomorphism. There has been recent interest in the application of immunohistochemical markers for the pre-operative diagnosis of follicular carcinoma, particularly galectin 3. A large European study suggested a positive predictive value of 92% and a diagnostic accuracy of 99% for galectin 3 positivity in predicting malignancy.[6] Though this might be helpful, it should be noted that focal positivity has been reported in a small proportion of follicular adenomas and in nodular goitre.[7] Although the patterns of staining are more focal, the nature of FNA sampling might give a false positive result. In addition, some follicular carcinomas have been reported negative for galectin 3.[8]

Follicular variant of papillary carcinoma may be recognised on cytology if the nuclear changes are pronounced. The smears show cells lying in sheets, cellular groups or microfollicles. Colloid is usually thin, with thick 'chewing gum' colloid less common than in the classic variant. The nuclei are elongated and show clearing of chromatin and thickening of the nuclear membrane; nuclear grooves and inclusions are said to be less common than in the classic variant. The presence of multinucleate giant cells is a factor in favour of the diagnosis of FVPC[9] and psammoma bodies may occasionally be found. In cases where a confident diagnosis can be made, these smears would be classified as Thy5. However, where the nuclear features are not prominent, the smear may be interpreted as a follicular neoplasm (Thy3) or as Thy4 if there is some clearing of chromatin and a thick nuclear membrane. To increase the sensitivity of detection of papillary carcinoma on FNA, one group has used reverse-transcriptase polymerase chain reaction (RT-PCR) for the specific ret/PTC gene re-arrangements that characterise a subset of these tumours.[10]

## NODULAR GOITRE

This disease develops as the result of absolute or relative deficiency of iodine intake. Goitre is defined as endemic in areas where more than 10% of the population is affected and sporadic when the incidence is less than that. Endemic goitre occurs in areas of iodine deficiency. Increased requirement for thyroid hormones, individual dietary insufficiency of iodine, ingestion of goitrogens and subclinical levels of dyshormonogenesis may be important in the pathogenesis of the sporadic form. The pathological features are a combination of hyperplastic and involutional change and nodule formation. The initial change is related to stimulation of secretion of thyroid hormones by pituitary thyroid stimulating hormone (TSH) in response to an increased demand for thyroxine. This results in thyroid hyperplasia, with the development of increased numbers of small follicles with little storage of colloid. The follicular cells are columnar and may show pleomorphism and mitotic activity. When the thyroid hormone levels reach normal, the gland undergoes a process of involution. The follicular cells become flattened and there is accumulation of colloid within the follicles. Eventually, after periods of stimulation and involution the thyroid comprises a mixture of hyperplastic and involutional change with areas of degeneration, haemorrhage and fibrosis. Some nodules may appear larger – dominant nodules. These may be nodules with extensive colloid accumulation and degeneration that are easily recognised on FNA, or hyperplastic nodules that histologically resemble follicular neoplasms. Some may be encapsulated. The question is whether to define them as adenomas or as nodules. In the context of overall nodularity, many pathologists would use the term 'adenomatoid nodule'. However, molecular analysis has shown that up to 70% of dominant nodules in nodular goitre are monoclonal, suggesting that they are neoplastic, while the remainder show a polyclonal pattern.[11] The specific classification is not important as long as after appropriate examination there are no features to indicate malignancy. Any nodules within a goitre that have a thick capsule should be processed as for a follicular neoplasm.

## FOLLICULAR ADENOMA

Follicular adenoma is the most common thyroid neoplasm (Fig. 1). It most often presents between 30–50 years of age with a female:male ratio of 20:1. It is

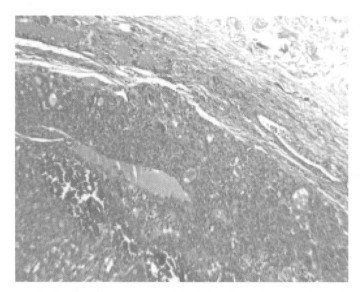

**Fig. 1** Follicular adenoma showing an expansile pattern of growth and a thin rather ill-formed capsule.

usually a single nodule with an expansile pattern of growth. Although they are described as encapsulated, the extent of capsule formation can vary. In some lesions, there is a well-formed fibrous capsule, though it is usually thin. Sometimes, the normal thyroid follicles adjacent to the tumour undergo atrophy, and the stroma condenses to form a pseudocapsule. In some cases, tumour cells abut directly onto normal thyroid parenchyma. However, even where they are in close contact with the normal follicles, an expansile pattern of growth is maintained and they do not infiltrate between follicles. A thick capsule is more often seen in follicular carcinoma.

In order to make the diagnosis, a proper assessment of the interface between the tumour and the normal gland is essential to rule out capsular or vascular invasion. It is suggested that lesions < 30 mm in diameter be processed in their entirety, and that larger lesions should have 8–10 blocks processed.[12,13] Follicular adenomas show a range of histological appearances. In some a microfollicular pattern predominates: in others there are mainly large colloid-filled follicles. Some tumours have a more solid or trabecular architecture. A mixed pattern may also be seen. These are of no clinical relevance. Most comprise small fairly uniform cells with round nuclei and evenly dispersed chromatin. There may be central degenerative change with hyalinisation or calcification, but these changes are more frequent in hyperplastic nodules. Mitotic activity is uncommon. In cases with marked nuclear atypia or mitotic activity, great care should be taken to rule out capsular or vascular invasion. Tumours with these features but no evidence of invasion are referred to as atypical adenomas. Most behave in a benign fashion. Areas of degeneration are often associated with pseudopapillary architecture, not to be confused with papillary carcinoma. There may also be some focal clearing of nuclei and this may cause the pathologist to consider a diagnosis of FVPC. In most cases it should be possible to make the distinction. The characteristic prominence of the nuclear membrane is not present and

5

nuclear grooves and inclusions are not usually seen. Immunostaining for cytokeratin (CK) 19 may show focal positivity, in contrast to the more wide-spread staining in FVPC. However, it should be noted that the threshold for interpreting nuclear features as characteristic of FVPC differs with individual pathologists. Follicles may become entrapped within the capsule in an adenoma but there is no penetration. Changes associated with FNA are discussed below.

Rare variants include adenolipoma, where the tumour cells are interspersed with mature adipose tissue. This probably represents adipose metaplasia. Clear cell and signet ring cell tumours are also described. An origin from thyroid follicular cells can be confirmed by immunopositivity for thyroglobulin and thyroid transcription factor-1 (TTF-1),[14] a nuclear protein important in regulating the transcription of the thyroglobulin gene. Care must be taken with all immunohistochemistry when biotin-based techniques are used as thyroid follicular cells may contain significant amounts of endogenous biotin.

## FOLLICULAR CARCINOMA

Follicular carcinoma accounts for 5–15% of all thyroid cancers. It is more common in women and presents on average about 10 years later than papillary carcinoma. It usually presents as a single 'cold' nodule. Occasional cases present as distant metastases, particularly in bone. On the basis of the extent of invasion, the tumour is subdivided into two categories – minimally invasive and widely invasive. Minimally invasive tumours are more common. These are diagnosed by the presence of microscopic capsular and/or vascular invasion. Widely invasive tumours can often be seen infiltrating the normal gland by naked eye examination. This diagnosis may also be applied when extensive vascular invasion is identified at microscopic level. It is important to make the distinction between the two, as the outcome varies significantly. The

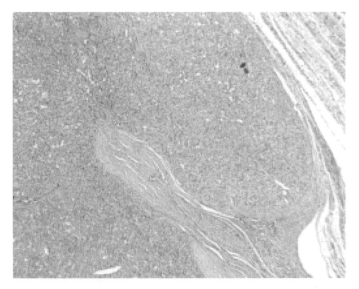

**Fig. 2** Minimally invasive follicular carcinoma showing capsular invasion. Note the blunt-ended break in the capsule and the mushroom-shaped extension of the tumour into the surrounding gland.

10-year survival rates for minimally invasive disease is 70–100% and for the widely invasive type, 25–45%.[15] Tumour-related deaths are more common in the widely invasive group, reported in 20–50% of cases, but in minimally invasive disease account for only 3% of deaths.[13,16]

Diagnosis of minimally invasive disease depends on the identification of capsular (Fig. 2) or vascular (Fig. 3) invasion, or both. There has been debate over the years as to the definitions of these two features. It is now generally accepted that tumour cells must penetrate the entire thickness of the capsule for the diagnosis of capsular invasion. This is usually associated with 'blunt end' breaks in the capsule and a 'streaming' or mushroom pattern of growth of tumour through the capsule. This is in contrast to the entrapment of follicles within the capsule of an adenoma where there is no impression of an active process of cell movement. It is important to appreciate that the penetrating tumour mass often stimulates the formation of a new capsule. This means that the tumour may have a dumbbell appearance, or that there is the impression of subdivision of a follicular tumour by a fragmented fibrous band. These appearances can be extremely difficult to interpret. Some pathologists would argue that malignant potential cannot be diagnosed on the basis of capsular invasion alone and would define these tumours as 'follicular neoplasms of undetermined malignant potential'. However, metastases have occurred in tumours where only capsular invasion has been identified.

Vascular invasion should be diagnosed only when tumour thrombi are attached to the wall of a medium-sized or large vessel, either within or outside the capsule, and are covered by endothelium. Tumour cells and vessels are often intermingled within the capsule and it can sometimes be difficult to determine whether this is true invasion. It may be necessary to use immunohistochemistry for an endothelial marker such as CD31 or CD34. Factor VIII-related antigen is not generally useful as it can be negative in vessels invaded by tumour. An

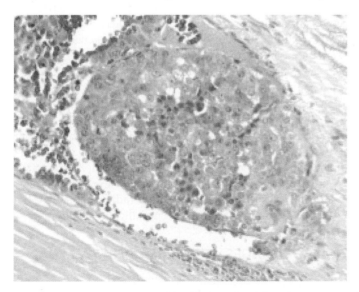

**Fig. 3** Minimally invasive follicular carcinoma showing vascular invasion. The tumour thrombus is attached to the vessel wall (upper right) and is covered by endothelium.

unusual feature that might also be misinterpreted as invasion is endothelial hyperplasia in capsular vessels. However, if this is seen, it should prompt a search for vascular invasion as it has usually been reported in carcinomas.[17]

Immunohistochemistry has been applied in an attempt to distinguish between benign and malignant lesions. Wide-spread strong positivity for galectin 3 supports a malignant diagnosis, but focal staining can be found in benign follicular lesions and not all carcinomas are positive.[18] HBME-1 also stains malignant lesions more commonly than benign.[19] Ancillary techniques such as ploidy analysis have no role in making the distinction between adenoma and carcinoma.

Widely invasive tumours are usually easy to define. Grossly, the tumour can be seen infiltrating the normal gland. Some have no evidence of a capsule, while others have a capsule with extensive capsular and vascular invasion.

## HÜRTHLE CELL (ONCOCYTIC) FOLLICULAR TUMOURS

Follicular tumours are defined as Hürthle cell when more than 75% of the tumour cells are oncocytic. Grossly, these are usually single nodules with a deep brown cut surface. They often undergo infarction following FNA, and it has been suggested that this may be related to their microvasculature, which is different from other thyroid tumours. A variety of growth patterns is seen in both benign and malignant tumours including microfollicular, macrofollicular, trabecular, solid and pseudopapillary architecture. Nuclear atypia and mitotic activity are common; some have suggested that where these features are marked, they signify malignant potential, but follow-up studies have refuted this. A category of atypical Hürthle cell adenoma has been proposed for such tumours and for those with spontaneous infarction or necrosis. A higher proportion (35%) of Hürthle cell tumours are malignant than of other follicular lesions. Trabecular and solid architecture are more common in Hürthle cell carcinomas.

The diagnosis of malignancy should be made solely on the basis of capsular and/or vascular invasion. Immunohistochemistry is not generally useful. Hürthle cell tumours stain positively for thyroglobulin, but the staining is usually weaker than in follicular lesions. Positivity for TTF-1 is variable.[20] Galectin 3 has been reported to stain up to 60% of carcinomas, but also gives positive staining of some adenomas.[21] A recent study has suggested that Hürthle cell carcinomas with a Ki-67 index > 5% show a more aggressive pattern of behaviour.[22]

Although the pathologist should approach the diagnosis of Hürthle cell tumours in the same manner as follicular tumours, there is increasing evidence that the molecular pathogenesis of these tumours differs from that of other follicular neoplasms.[23,24] This may to some extent explain the differences in behaviour. Hürthle cell tumours rarely take up radio-iodine: lymph node and distant metastases are more common than in follicular carcinoma.

## HISTOLOGICAL CHANGES AFTER PRE-OPERATIVE FNA CYTOLOGY

Alterations in histology caused by pre-operative FNA are increasingly recognised by pathologists in surgical specimens (Fig. 4). Some of these cause problems in diagnosis. Sometimes a needle track is obvious, with haemor-

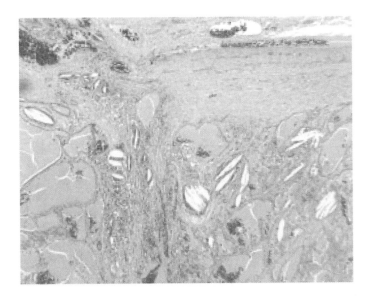

**Fig. 4** Follicular adenoma showing post-FNA changes. There is a focus of disruption and distortion of the capsule, with entrapment of follicles. This is associated with obvious evidence of haemorrhage and tissue damage within the tumour, as seen by the cholesterol clefts and fibrosis. At high power, there were significant numbers of foamy and haemosiderin-laden macrophages.

rhage, granulation tissue and haemosiderin-laden macrophages. Cholesterol crystals may be present. The cells in the adjacent follicles may show some enlargement and atypia. There may be distortion or disruption of the capsule where the needle has passed through. The capsular changes may raise the question of invasion, particularly when there is active fibrogenesis with follicles in the capsule. The pattern is linear, however, in contrast to the 'mushroom' pattern of growth usually seen with true invasion and the breaks in the capsule do not have the characteristic blunt ends. Haemosiderin-laden macrophages are common in the vicinity of a needle-track. Several weeks or months after FNA, small foci of squamous metaplasia may be seen in the area of the capsule. It is important not to interpret these as squamous cell carcinoma. Spindle cell nodules have also been described[25] and these should not be confused with a de-differentiated component of the tumour.

Tumour infarction can also be seen; Hürthle cell tumours are particularly susceptible to this. When the whole tumour is infarcted, it can be difficult to make a diagnosis. Papillary endothelial hyperplasia has been described in the centre of aspirated nodules. This may be related to thrombosis and recanalisation of vessels after FNA.

## FOLLICULAR VARIANT OF PAPILLARY CARCINOMA

This is the next commonest variant to the classic variant of papillary carcinoma. There is follicular architecture but the cells lining the follicles have the cytological features of papillary carcinoma (Fig. 5). Where a mixed pattern

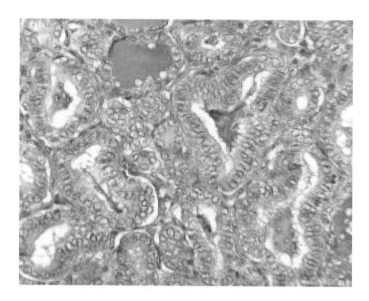

**Fig. 5** Follicular variant of papillary carcinoma. The follicles show some irregularity and are lined by cells with the characteristic nuclear appearance of papillary carcinoma. Some of the follicles contain multinucleate giant cells.

of classic papillary and follicular architecture is present, the tumour should be classified as a classic variant. Most of these tumours are not encapsulated or have a poorly formed capsule. Prominent fibrous bands may extend between the tumour cells. The follicles are often of irregular shape with abortive attempts to produce papillae. There may also be interconnections between neighbouring follicles.[26] The cells are larger than normal follicular cells and have an oval or elongated shape. The nuclei are defined as 'optically clear' and show clearing of chromatin and a prominent nuclear membrane (Fig. 4). Nuclear grooves and pseudo-inclusions reflect invagination of the cytoplasm into the nucleus. There is heaping up of nuclei, with what has been described as a 'basket of eggs' appearance. Psammoma bodies may be present. The presence of multinucleate cells in the lumens of the follicles is another clue to diagnosis. These have a histiocytic phenotype.[27]

Where these features are pronounced and present throughout the tumour, the diagnosis is easy. In some tumours, the changes are more focal and distinction has to be made from follicular tumours or hyperplastic nodules. This can be difficult. A panel of antibodies has been proposed. These include antibodies to cytokeratin 19 (CK19), HBME-1 and RET. In a series of 84 cases, 57% were positive for CK19, 45% for HBME-1 and 63% for RET protein. Only seven cases were negative for all three proteins.[28] Strong diffuse staining for cytokeratin 19 is usually seen in the areas with nuclear changes with weaker staining in the rest of the tumour (Fig. 6). This contrasts with the focal reactivity that can be seen in follicular tumours. Immunostaining with the antibodies to RET protein can be difficult. In a few cases, it is extremely difficult to be sure of the diagnosis, and even endocrine pathologists will disagree as to how to categorise the lesion. It may be appropriate to say that the diagnosis of FVPC cannot be fully excluded. The development of multidisciplinary teams will permit discussion of how to proceed in these cases.

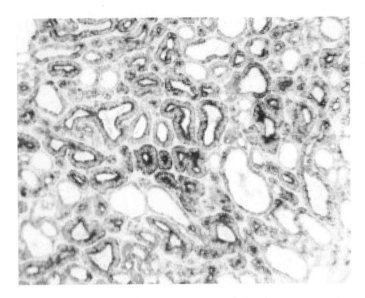

**Fig. 6** Follicular variant of papillary carcinoma. This medium-power view shows strong diffuse staining for cytokeratin 19.

There are a number of patterns of growth of FVPC in the gland and it is important to recognise these as the behaviour may differ. The diffuse type of FVPC invade widely.[29] It forms multiple nodules throughout the gland and is commonly associated with lymph node and distant metastases. Other FVPCs are encapsulated and have a good prognosis. Another type is the macro-follicular variant.[30] This tumour appears also to have a good outcome. On low power, foci of tumour resemble hyperplastic nodules; the differential diagnosis may include macrofollicular adenoma and nodular goitre. The recognition of the nuclear features is important in making these distinctions.

## FOLLICULAR VARIANT OF MEDULLARY CARCINOMA

Medullary carcinomas can have a range of appearances and sometimes contain scattered follicular structures. Some of these are formed by tumour cells and others are entrapped normal follicles. Rarely, the predominant pattern is follicular. Immunostaining will show positivity for calcitonin in the cells in the follicular structures if they are tumour cells, with negative staining for thyroglobulin. In contrast, normal follicles can be identified by positivity for thyroglobulin.

## MIXED FOLLICULAR AND MEDULLARY CARCINOMA

This is a rare group of tumours. There is evidence of both follicular and C-cell differentiation. They have been referred to as mixed, composite or inter-mediate tumours. In some, the individual tumour cells show immuno-positivity for both calcitonin and thyroglobulin,[31] while in others there seem to be two individual populations. It has been suggested that they may arise from

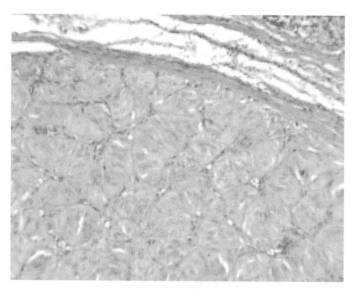

**Fig. 7** Hyalinising trabecular tumour. This medium-power view shows the trabecular arrangement and the elongated cells characteristic of this tumour.

stem cells of the ultimobranchial body or that they represent collision tumours. The latter explanation would be a possibility where two individual tumour components are identified (composite tumours) and recent molecular studies lend support to this concept.[32] However, this theory does not adequately explain the expression of calcitonin and thyroglobulin in the same tumour cell.

## HYALINISING TRABECULAR TUMOUR

This is a rare tumour that was first defined by Carney as hyalinising trabecular adenoma[33] though it had been described earlier. The clinical behaviour of the original series was benign, thus the term adenoma. More recent reports suggest that there is a malignant counterpart and these lesions are now defined as hyalinising trabecular tumours: the expected behaviour is defined on the basis of capsular and vascular invasion. It is an encapsulated lesion derived from follicular cells comprising trabeculae of elongated cells around vascular channels surrounded by matrix (Fig. 7). The matrix may be hyalinised or show calcification. The nuclei may be elongated and have grooves and inclusions. Psammoma bodies may be present. Yellow intracytoplasmic inclusions have been described: these contain lipid, glycosaminoglycan and proteoglycan and are consistent with giant lysosomes. They are present in most hyalinising trabecular tumours, but are not specific as they may occasionally be found in follicular adenomas. Morphological changes resembling this tumour can be seen focally in some follicular adenomas and hyperplastic nodules.

Their histogenesis has been unclear. The overall arrangement of the cells resembles medullary carcinoma and paraganglioma and the lesion has also been named 'paraganglioma-like adenoma of thyroid (PLAT)'. None of these tumours express calcitonin and all show immunopositivity for thyroglobulin, suggesting an origin from follicular cells. Focal positivity for general neuroendocrine

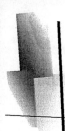
# How to......

## Access the library catalogue
### View items in local NHS Trust libraries

1. Visit **www.base-library.nhs.uk/nhs_libraries.asp**
2. Click on the University Hospital Birmingham NHS Trust link.
3. Scroll down to the end of the Queen Elizabeth Hospital Library details, and click on the LMS Link.

## Set your own unique PIN
### Check and renew your loans using
### your library card barcode and unique PIN

To set your own unique PIN:
1. Click on the 'My Account' link in the yellow menu bar.
2. Click on the 'User PIN Change' icon.
3. Enter your library card barcode into the 'User ID' box, and '1111' into the 'PIN box.
4. Enter your own unique PIN twice, in the '...new PIN' boxes, and click on the 'Change PIN' button.

If you experience any difficulties, then please contact:
QEH Library: ext.8266 OR SOH Library: ext.52325

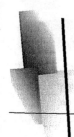

**Once you have re-registered with the library, you will be able to borrow items from the following Trust Libraries:**

Birmingham Children's Hospital
Birmingham Women's Hospital
City Hospital
Good Hope Hospital
Heartlands Hospital
Highcroft Hospital
Queen Elizabeth Hospital
Queen Elizabeth Psychiatric Hospital
Reaside Clinic
Sandwell Hospital
Selly Oak Hospital
Solihull Hospital
South Birmingham PCT, Moseley Hall Hospital

**Contact details and opening hours for the above can be found at:**
www.base-library.nhs.uk/nhs_libraries.asp

Base-Library
1st base for quality e-resources

University Hospital **NHS**
Birmingham
NHS Foundation Trust

UHB TRUST LIBRARIES

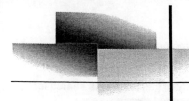

## USING THE LIBRARY CATALOGUE

**UHB Trust intranet -**
http://uhbhome
(Trust username and password required)
Departments
Library
Our Services
UHB Online Catalogue
**Internet -**
http://www.bhsn.sirsi.ltd.uk/uhtbin/webcat
(Simply click on the 'Login' button)

You can now view books and other materials held in local NHS Trust libraries. Click on **Library Opening Hours** on the homepage to check which libraries you can use. Click on a specific library for their details.

Login from the homepage, using your library card barcode as **User ID** and your unique **PIN** to access all the features of the online catalogue.

To create your unique PIN, click on **My Account** in the top yellow menu bar. Click on the **User PIN Change** icon, and enter your library card barcode as **User ID** and **1111** for the **PIN**. Enter your own unique PIN twice, in the ...**new PIN** boxes, and click on the **Change PIN** button.

## SEARCHING

•Enter your search term in the search box on the home page.

•From the drop-down menu next to the search box, you can choose to search for a **title** or **author** only.

•From the drop-down menu beneath the search box, you can choose to search for items at a specific library, e.g. **Queen Elizabeth Hospital Library**.

•Click on the **Search** button.

## SEARCH RESULTS

•The results of your search show the title, edition, author, and year of publication.

**NB:** The shelfmark, e.g. **QS 4**, is where the item is shelved in only one of the libraries, if you have searched all libraries.

•To check which libraries hold the item, where it is shelved, and whether it is available for loan, click on the **Details** button to the left of the title.

•The **Location** column shows whether a copy is **Available** (for loan) or **Reference** (for use in the home library). Where there is a date, this indicates when that copy is due for return to the library.

## RESERVING

**NB:** Items cannot be requested from other libraries until 2005.

•To reserve a copy, click on **Place Hold** in the left-hand box.

•From the drop-down menu, select the library you want to collect the item from, and click on the **Place Hold** button.

•You will be notified when the item is available for collection.

**If you want further details on all the features of the online catalogue,
please contact: QEH Library: ext.8266 OR SOH Library: ext.52325**

markers has been described in some raising the possibility of dual differentiation. The relation to papillary carcinoma has been most widely debated. The nuclear features resemble those of papillary carcinoma and psammoma bodies are sometimes present. Papillary carcinoma can be found in the thyroid gland in about one-third of cases of hyalinising trabecular tumour and may co-exist in the same nodule. Immunohistochemical data are inconsistent. Some have reported positivity for CK19; others have found this to be negative. Recent studies have shown ret/PTC arrangements in some of these lesions, suggesting that they are a variant of papillary carcinoma.[34,35] However, not all cases show these changes and hyalinising trabecular tumours may represent a spectrum of neoplasia.

## CONCLUSIONS

Molecular analysis is now clarifying the pathways in the development of the various types of thyroid tumour.[36] Interestingly, unlike other solid tumours, translocations occur in follicular tumours and papillary carcinoma. Follicular carcinoma shows a PAX8–PPARγ fusion,[37] and papillary carcinoma has a range of RET re-arrangements.[38] These findings are not yet translating into useful diagnostic tests though they may come in the next few years. The mainstay of diagnosis remains the histological examination of appropriately sampled tissue backed up by immunohistochemistry where appropriate.

---

### Points of best practice

- All thyroid tumours should be dealt with by a multidisciplinary team that includes a pathologist.

- Fine needle aspiration cytology should be the first line investigation of a thyroid lump.

- It is essential to sample the tumour/normal interface widely in follicular tumours to assess capsular and vascular invasion. Tumours less than 3 cm in diameter should be processed in their entirety and larger lesions should have 8–10 blocks taken.

- In follicular lesions, vascular invasion should be diagnosed only when tumour thrombus is present in medium-to-large vessels lying within or outwith the capsule. The presence of tumour cells in intratumoural vessels is not included.

- Immunohistochemistry for galectin 3 may be helpful in diagnosing malignancy, but is not an absolute predictor.

- It is important to identify Hürthle cell tumours because of their different behavioural characteristics.

- Follicular variant of papillary carcinoma is characterised by optically clear nuclei. Irregular follicular shape and the presence of intrafollicular multinucleate cells may help to raise suspicions.

## References

1. British Thyroid Association. *Guidelines for the Management of Thyroid Cancer in Adults.* London: The Royal College of Physicians, 2002.
2. Hamberger B, Gharib H, Melton 3rd LJ, Goellner JR, Zinsmeister AR. Fine-needle aspiration biopsy of thyroid nodules. Impact on thyroid practice and cost of care. *Am J Med* 1982; **73**: 381–384.
3. Hundahl SA, Cady B, Cunningham MP *et al.* Initial results from a prospective cohort study of 5583 cases of thyroid carcinoma treated in the United States during 1996. US and German Thyroid Cancer Study Group. An American College of Surgeons Commission on Cancer Patient Care Evaluation study. *Cancer* 2000; **89**: 202–217.
4. Chen H, Dudley NE, Westra WH, Sadler GP, Udelsman R. Utilization of fine-needle aspiration in patients undergoing thyroidectomy at two academic centers across the Atlantic. *World J Surg* 2003; **27**: 208–211.
5. Goellner JR. Problems and pitfalls in thyroid cytology. *Monogr Pathol* 1997; **39**: 75–93.
6. Bartolazzi A, Gasbarri A, Papotti M *et al.* Application of an immunodiagnostic method for improving preoperative diagnosis of nodular thyroid lesions. *Lancet* 2001; **357**: 1644–1650.
7. Beesley MF, McLaren KM. Cytokeratin 19 and galectin-3 immunohistochemistry in the differential diagnosis of solitary thyroid nodules. *Histopathology* 2002; **41**: 236–243.
8. Herrmann ME, LiVolsi VA, Pasha TL, Roberts SA, Wojcik EM, Baloch ZW. Immunohistochemical expression of galectin-3 in benign and malignant thyroid lesions. *Arch Pathol Lab Med* 2002; **126**: 710–713.
9. Tsou PL, Hsiao YL, Chang TC. Multinucleated giant cells in fine needle aspirates. Can they help differentiate papillary thyroid cancer from benign nodular goiter? *Acta Cytol* 2002; **46**: 823–827.
10. Cheung CC, Carydis B, Ezzat S, Bedard YC, Asa SL. Analysis of ret/PTC gene rearrangements refines the fine needle aspiration diagnosis of thyroid cancer. *J Clin Endocrinol Metab* 2001; **86**: 2187–2190.
11. Baloch ZW, LiVolsi VA. Clonality in thyroid nodules: the hyperplasia-neoplasia sequence. *Endocr Pathol* 1998; **9**: 287–292.
12. Franssila KO, Ackerman LV, Brown CL, Hedinger CE. Follicular carcinoma. *Semin Diagn Pathol* 1985; **2**: 101–122.
13. Lang W, Choritz H, Hundeshagen H. Risk factors in follicular thyroid carcinomas. A retrospective follow-up study covering a 14-year period with emphasis on morphological findings. *Am J Surg Pathol* 1986; **10**: 246–255.
14. Katoh R, Kawaoi A, Miyagi E *et al.* Thyroid transcription factor-1 in normal, hyperplastic, and neoplastic follicular thyroid cells examined by immunohistochemistry and nonradioactive *in situ* hybridization. *Mod Pathol* 2000; **13**: 570–576.
15. Rosai J, Carcangiu ML, DeLellis RA. *Tumors of the Thyroid Gland*, 3rd series edn. Washington, DC: Armed Forces Institute of Pathology, 1992.
16. Woolner LB. Thyroid carcinoma: pathologic classification with data on prognosis. *Semin Nucl Med* 1971; **1**: 481–502.
17. Tse LL, Chan I, Chan JK. Capsular intravascular endothelial hyperplasia: a peculiar form of vasoproliferative lesion associated with thyroid carcinoma. *Histopathology* 2001; **39**: 463–468.
18. Cvejic D, Savin S, Paunovic I, Tatic S, Havelka M, Sinadinovic J. Immunohistochemical localization of galectin-3 in malignant and benign human thyroid tissue. *Anticancer Res* 1998; **18**: 2637–2641.
19. Miettinen M, Karkkainen P. Differential reactivity of HBME-1 and CD15 antibodies in benign and malignant thyroid tumours. Preferential reactivity with malignant tumours. *Virchows Arch* 1996; **429**: 213–219.
20. Bejarano PA, Nikiforov YE, Swenson ES, Biddinger PW. Thyroid transcription factor-1, thyroglobulin, cytokeratin 7, and cytokeratin 20 in thyroid neoplasms. *Appl Immunohistochem Mol Morphol* 2000; **8**: 189–194.
21. Nascimento MC, Bisi H, Alves VA, Longatto-Filho A, Kanamura CT, Medeiros-Neto G. Differential reactivity for galectin-3 in Hürthle cell adenomas and carcinomas. *Endocr Pathol* 2001; **12**: 275–279.

22. Hoos A, Stojadinovic A, Singh B *et al.* Clinical significance of molecular expression profiles of Hürthle cell tumors of the thyroid gland analyzed via tissue microarrays. *Am J Pathol* 2002; **160**: 175–183.
23. Zedenius J, Wallin G, Svensson A *et al.* Allelotyping of follicular thyroid tumors. *Hum Genet* 1995; **96**: 27–32.
24. Segev DL, Saji M, Phillips GS *et al.* Polymerase chain reaction-based microsatellite polymorphism analysis of follicular and Hürthle cell neoplasms of the thyroid. *J Clin Endocrinol Metab* 1998; **83**: 2036–2042.
25. Baloch ZW, Wu H, LiVolsi VA. Post-fine-needle aspiration spindle cell nodules of the thyroid (PSCNT). *Am J Clin Pathol* 1999; **111**: 70–74.
26. Bell CD, Coire C, Treger T, Volpe R, Baumal R, Fornasier VL. The 'dark nucleus' and disruptions of follicular architecture: possible new histological aids for the diagnosis of the follicular variant of papillary carcinoma of the thyroid. *Histopathology* 2001; **39**: 33–42.
27. Tabbara SO, Acoury N, Sidawy MK. Multinucleated giant cells in thyroid neoplasms. A cytologic, histologic and immunohistochemical study. *Acta Cytol* 1996; **40**: 1184–1188.
28. Cheung CC, Ezzat S, Freeman JL, Rosen IB, Asa SL. Immunohistochemical diagnosis of papillary thyroid carcinoma. *Mod Pathol* 2001; **14**: 338–342.
29. Ivanova R, Soares P, Castro P, Sobrinho-Simoes M. Diffuse (or multinodular) follicular variant of papillary thyroid carcinoma: a clinicopathologic and immunohistochemical analysis of ten cases of an aggressive form of differentiated thyroid carcinoma. *Virchows Arch* 2002; **440**: 418–424.
30. Albores-Saavedra J, Gould E, Vardaman C, Vuitch F. The macrofollicular variant of papillary thyroid carcinoma: a study of 17 cases. *Hum Pathol* 1991; **22**: 1195–1205.
31. Holm R, Sobrinho-Simoes M, Nesland JM, Johannessen JV. Concurrent production of calcitonin and thyroglobulin by the same neoplastic cells. *Ultrastruct Pathol* 1986; **10**: 241–248.
32. Papotti M, Volante M, Komminoth P, Sobrinho-Simoes M, Bussolati G. Thyroid carcinomas with mixed follicular and C-cell differentiation patterns. *Semin Diagn Pathol* 2000; **17**: 109–119.
33. Carney JA, Ryan J, Goellner JR. Hyalinizing trabecular adenoma of the thyroid gland. *Am J Surg Pathol* 1987; **11**: 583–591.
34. Papotti M, Volante M, Giuliano A *et al.* RET/PTC activation in hyalinizing trabecular tumors of the thyroid. *Am J Surg Pathol* 2000; **24**: 1615–1621.
35. Cheung CC, Boerner SL, MacMillan CM, Ramyar L, Asa SL. Hyalinizing trabecular tumor of the thyroid: a variant of papillary carcinoma proved by molecular genetics. *Am J Surg Pathol* 2000; **24**: 1622–1626.
36. Kroll TG. Molecular rearrangements and morphology in thyroid cancer. *Am J Pathol* 2002; **160**: 1941–1944.
37. Nikiforova MN, Biddinger PW, Caudill CM, Kroll TG, Nikiforov YE. PAX8-PPARgamma rearrangement in thyroid tumors: RT-PCR and immunohistochemical analyses. *Am J Surg Pathol* 2002; **26**: 1016–1023.
38. Tallini G, Asa SL. RET oncogene activation in papillary thyroid carcinoma. *Adv Anat Pathol* 2001; **8**: 345–354.

*Esther J. Millward, Mark K. Heatley*

**2**

# Cytokeratin immuno-staining profiles in diagnostic pathology

Cytokeratins (CKs) are intermediate filament proteins, a group of proteins that derives its name from the fact that their diameter is between that of actin and tubulin, the protein types together with which they form the cytoskeleton. There are 8 basic (CK 1–8) and 12 acidic cytokeratins (CK 9–20). Cytokeratins typically occur in epithelial cells but also occur in other cell types.

Antibodies to cytokeratin intermediate filament proteins have been used for many years to verify the epithelial origin of poorly differentiated carcinoma and to identify small volumes of tumour, often at metastatic sites including lymph nodes and meninges. More recently, the development of antibodies which react to specific cytokeratins in tissue that has been fixed in formalin and embedded in paraffin wax has permitted investigators to examine the cytokeratin profile of lesions including benign and malignant tumours. In a recent review, Chu and Weiss[1] used these data to compile tables indicating the frequency with which each of the 20 cytokeratins is encountered in carcinomas of the major body sites with an aggregate experience ranging from a single case (CK 7 positivity and CK 20 negativity in Müllerian duct carcinoma) to 956 cases (an investigation of CK 20 expression in lobular and ductal carcinoma of the breast). This chapter examines the opportunities provided by these more specific anticytokeratin antibodies in diagnostic anatomical pathology.

## CYTOKERATIN PROFILES

### CYTOKERATIN PROFILES IN THE DIAGNOSIS OF METASTATIC DISEASE

The presence of a metastatic tumour deposit with either no apparent primary site or with several possible sites of origin provides a major clinical problem

**Dr Esther J. Millward** BSc MBChB
SpR Histopathology, St James's University Hospital, The Leeds Teaching Hospitals NHS Trust.

**Dr Mark K. Heatley**
Consultant Gynaecological Histopathologist, St James's University Hospital, The Leeds Teaching Hospitals NHS Trust, Beckett Street, Leeds LS9 7TF, UK.  Tel/Fax: +44 113 2067133

especially given the different therapeutic regimens that are now used for neoplasms that have originated at different primary sites. In many instances, this is elucidated using a combination of clinical and radiological data or by identifying a morphological pattern (such as Orphan Annie nuclei in papillary thyroid tumours) or protein expression by immunohistochemistry (such as PSA expression in prostatic carcinoma) that is characteristic of a primary tumour. Most tumours, however, lack such specific features and the cytokeratin profile has been advanced as a means of predicting the likely primary site of metastases.

## PRESERVATION OF CYTOKERATIN PROFILES

Ronnett et al.[2] examined the expression of CK 7 and CK 20 in a series of appendiceal carcinomas with several histomorphological patterns and their ovarian metastases and found a similar spectrum of reaction in the primary and secondary tumours. The diagnostic use of the paper by Ronnett et al.,[2] which appears to demonstrate that in some gastrointestinal tumours at least metastatic carcinomas maintain the cytokeratin profile of their primary lesion, was illustrated by Young and Hart[3] who used CK 7 and CK 20 expression to confirm that five ovarian tumours were metastases from colon rather than primary endometrioid adenocarcinoma of ovary. They extended their panel by including antibodies to carcino-embryonic antigen (CEA) and Ca 125. (This antibody profile has been used to confirm that an adenocarcinoma located in the colon arose in a focus of endometriosis and did not represent a primary colonic carcinoma.) In Paget's disease of the nipple, the intra-epidermal tumour cells in most cases contained CK 7 (35/37 cases), one of the negative cases being a CK 7-negative carcinoma.[4] Although it is suggested that during metastasis tumours retain their cytokeratin profiles,[5] aside from these studies papers comparing the cytokeratin expression of primary tumours and their known metastases are scarce and the assumption that the two are reliably the same has a slender evidence base. Studies in which cytokeratin expression in primary and metastatic tumours has been compared have found discrepancies though in these studies the biopsy fragments have been small or cytokeratin staining focal.[6]

## CYTOKERATIN PROFILES IN PRIMARY LESIONS ARISING AT DIFFERENT SITES

Assuming that this apparent preservation of immunoprofile in metastatic lesions applies to other than gynaecological practice, it should be remembered that there may be some overlap of immunostaining in tumours that have originated at different primary sites but have metastasised to the site under consideration – occasional primary mucinous tumours of ovary show the immunophenotype usually associated with colorectal tumours.[7] This particular problem was addressed by Lagendyk et al.[8] who examined the use of a panel of antibodies and found that CK 7 and CEA provided the best combination of markers to discriminate between carcinoma of bowel and ovary. Even so, one of their 57 test cases would have been misclassified had the diagnosis depended on using these two markers in isolation. In a later series, the same authors[8] studied a larger group of tumours that included 55 primary and 64 metastatic breast carcinomas and concluded that the addition of antibodies to oestrogen receptors and gross cystic disease fluid protein 15 permitted 89% of metastatic colorectal, 72% of metastatic breast and 96% of metastatic ovarian carcinomas to be identified correctly. These results indicate that immunohistochemical studies should be interpreted in the light of the clinical history and morphology of the tumours.

This is further demonstrated by the finding that CK 7 and CK 20 expression may be of value in distinguishing a colorectal metastasis in the liver from a cholangiocarcinoma especially if the lesion is peripherally located;[9] as this depends on the site of the metastatic lesion being known, it re-inforces the concept that interpretation of the results of differential cytokeratin reactions depends on an appropriate correlation with the clinical and histological findings.

## CYTOKERATIN PROFILES SHARED BY PRIMARY TUMOURS OF AND METASTATIC TUMOURS TO THE SAME GIVEN SITE

Similar cytokeratin profiles to those of primary tumours that have given rise to the metastases at a site of interest can occur in tumours that occur as primary malignancies at that site, even if they are of a different histological type. For example, though antibodies to CK 5/6 have been used to distinguish between primary pulmonary adenocarcinomas infiltrating pleura (which are mostly CK 5/6-negative) and mesotheliomas (CK 5/6-positive), CK 5/6 expression is also seen in adenocarcinoma originating at non-pulmonary sites and metastasising to thoracic organs. Whilst primary pulmonary adenocarcinoma may be differentiated from mesothelioma by the antibody to CK 5/6, this antibody alone cannot be used to differentiate between a mesothelioma and an adenocarcinoma metastatic from one of these other sites[10] or from a primary squamous cell carcinoma of the lung, which may also be CK 5/6-positive. These findings were largely confirmed by Carella et al.[11] who advocated the use of a panel that included BerEp4, calretinin and CEA to distinguish these lesions. To re-inforce this point, three lesions that occur commonly and which are morphologically similar are malignant mesothelioma (53% of cases positive for CK 5/6), primary serous papillary carcinoma of the peritoneum (0% positive for CK 5/6), and metastatic serous papillary ovarian carcinoma (25% positive for CK 5/6). Calretinin and BerEp4 antibodies were again judged to be both more sensitive and specific in distinguishing these lesions.[12] It must be emphasised that these series included examples of malignancies which did not follow these rules.

The expansion of an antibody panel seems to be useful especially if it is tailored to the clinical and histopathological features of the lesion. CK 14 expression was identified in 90% of cases of squamous cell carcinoma regardless of grade and exclusively in areas of squamous differentiation in 4% of cases of adenocarcinoma.[13] This finding could be of value to distinguish between poorly differentiated squamous carcinoma of lung and primary or metastatic adenocarcinoma. This study was based on the morphological identification of squamous differentiation using H&E stained sections; but squamous differentiation has been shown to be more common than is morphologically obvious on immunohistochemical investigation with antibodies to involucrin.[14]

An antibody to CK 14 was also useful in identifying oncocytic tumours, all of which were CK 14-positive.[13] Cytokeratin antibodies were found to be the most effective means of distinguishing between renal cell carcinoma (8% 34 βE 12-positive) and ovarian clear cell carcinoma (100% 34 βE 12-positive) though ideally a panel which also included antibodies to Ca 125, vimentin, oestrogen and progesterone receptors should be used.[15]

## DISTINCTION BETWEEN *IN SITU* AND INVASIVE DISEASE

Traditionally, this distinction has depended on the finding that CK 5 and CK 14 highlight basal and myoepithelial cells. Use of antibodies to demonstrate that the basement membrane is intact or has been breached distinguishes *in situ* from invasive neoplasia. Antibodies to CK 14 were found to be less valuable than those to actin in distinguishing tubular carcinoma of breast from non-neoplastic conditions[16] and invasive cancer from *in situ* carcinoma of breast.[17] In a short series of 30 prostate needle biopsies, CK 5/6 was found to be more sensitive than antibody 34 βE 12 at differentiating between non-neoplastic and malignant prostate glands.[18]

As well as demonstrating whether there is an intact basal or myoepithelial cell layer, the cytokeratin profile in the epithelial proliferation itself may be helpful diagnostically and a number of studies have compared the reaction to cytokeratin antibodies in morphologically similar lesions. Hyalinizing trabecular adenoma is not usually reactive for 34 βE 12 or CK 19 whereas papillary thyroid carcinoma usually shows an intense reaction to both.[19] Although this study was carried out to establish that these lesions were distinct biological entities, the results may assist non-specialist pathologists in the diagnosis of a difficult thyroid lesion.

Immunohistochemistry has been of less use in elucidating other diagnostic challenges: for example, a battery of immunohistochemical stains that included antibodies to CK 18 and CK 19 was not found to be of use in distinguishing between atypical adenomatous hyperplasia and well-differentiated hepatocellular carcinoma. CK 19 was of some use in the differential diagnosis of hepatocellular carcinoma from cholangicarcinoma.[20]

Several studies have demonstrated that the distribution of immunostaining is of diagnostic importance and not simply whether there is a positive or negative reaction pattern. CK 19 expression was found not to be confined to papillary thyroid carcinoma in a study comparing its occurrence with that in follicular adenoma, but the staining reaction in the carcinomas tended to be more intense and diffuse than with follicular adenoma in which staining tended to be located in the cells lining cystic follicles or at the periphery of the nodule.[21]

## *IN SITU* AND REACTIVE, NON-NEOPLASTIC DISEASE

Cytokeratin antibodies have been found to be of some value in distinguishing reactive, non-neoplastic diseases from pre-invasive cancer. McKenney *et al.*[22] found that patchy CK 20 expression was confined to the umbrella cells of normal ureteric epithelium and urothelium showing reactive atypia: intense positivity was present in urothelial carcinoma *in situ*.

One of the most exciting studies in terms of prognostic and therapeutic potential has been in predicting the biological behaviour of lesions that previously would have been managed identically. Harnden et al.[23] found that there was no recurrence in 10 patients with non-invasive papillary bladder tumours and a normal CK 20 distribution: 30 of the 41 patients (73%) with abnormal CK 20 expression in a morphologically similar non-invasive tumour developed a recurrence within a median of 6 months In this study, CK 20 immunostaining in superficial and occasional intermediate cells throughout the tumour was regarded as normal; any staining greater than this was considered abnormal. These findings may be of especial value to the non-specialist when dealing with suboptimal or abraided tissues.

In the breast, CK 5/6 expression may be a means of distinguishing between non-neoplastic, reactive lesions in which the epithelial cells were CK 5/6-positive and atypical hyperplasia and *in situ* carcinoma, in which the hyperplastic and neoplastic cells were CK 5/6-negative. An appreciation of morphology is still essential: reactive cells in an otherwise neoplastic proliferation can express CK 5/6 and lead to confusion and misdiagnosis.

## REACTIVE VERSUS INVASIVE CARCINOMA

Cytokeratin profiles may be helpful in confirming a diagnosis in reactive conditions and benign neoplasia which may be confused with malignant disease. For example, atypical nephrogenic metaplasia[24] of the prostate is 34 βE 12-positive whereas invasive prostatic carcinoma with which it may be confused is 34 βE 12-negative.

There is a need here for caution. Similar cytokeratin profiles occur in non-neoplastic, benign and malignant lesions at some sites.[30] Occasionally, unexpected reactions may occur such as breast carcinoma that reacts for CK 14, a protein usually expressed in myoepithelial cells.

## USE OF CYTOKERATINS IN DISTINGUISHING AMONG DIFFERENT REACTIVE CONDITIONS

Cytokeratin profiles have been studied less in non-neoplastic reactive conditions than in neoplastic ones and may be of value in determining the embryological origin of normal structures.[25] Ormsby et al.[26] examined CK 7 and CK 20 expression in Barrett's oesophagus and suggested that these antibodies might be useful in distinguishing Barrett's oesophagus from intestinal metaplasia of the cardia of the stomach. Most cases of Barrett's oesophagus (63/65) were associated with CK 20 staining in superficial glands and CK 7 staining in the deep and superficial glands. There was no staining for either CK 20 or CK 7 in any of the biopsies from 24 patients with intestinal metaplasia of the stomach.

Goldstein et al.[27] studied the morphological features in liver biopsies from patients with primary biliary cirrhosis (PBC) and autoimmune hepatitis (AIH). The biopsies selected for study were not considered to be diagnostic and the diagnoses were based on clinical and serological findings. Three-quarters of the cases of PBC had CK 7-positive periportal hepatocytes, which were present in fewer than 10% of portal tracts from 2 of the 16 patients with AIH. These studies provide observational data that justify further investigation of the value of cytokeratin antibodies in the diagnosis of reactive diseases.

## USE OF CYTOKERATINS IN TYPING CARCINOMA

The distinction of common carcinomas is easily achieved in most cases using H&E staining but the differing immunophenotypes of some cancers may help in refining a diagnosis. Lehr *et al.*[28] found that the cells of lobular carcinoma of the breast had a ring-like perinuclear distribution of CK 8 and ductal carcinoma had a diffuse cytoplasmic reaction, with moulding where cell borders came in contact. They considered that this was a means of distinguishing ductal carcinoma which had an Indian-file pattern from lobular carcinoma. This work may provide an explanation for the biological behaviour of these tumours as the authors also found that cadherin E was clearly positive with ductal carcinoma and negative with lobular carcinoma. The diagnostic significance of the staining distribution was also shown by Liberman and Weidener[29] who found that 91% of papillary carcinoma of thyroid, including the follicular variant, showed a strong patchy reaction for 34 βE 12. Only 20% of follicular neoplasms reacted and in contrast showed a weak, diffuse reaction pattern.

## LIMITATIONS OF THE USE OF CYTOKERATINS IN TYPING PRIMARY MALIGNANCY

In the past there has been a tendency to present the results of cytokeratin antibody staining of tumours in terms that imply that a particular tumour is either positive or negative for that cytokeratin. This has resulted in the misconception, especially amongst non-pathologists, that a cytokeratin profile examined in isolation permits the origin of a tumour to be confidently determined even though the panel may be limited to one or two antibodies. In the tables which they prepared by aggregating the findings of other authors' series, Chu and Weiss[1] had the foresight to present the actual percentage of each tumour type. Confidence intervals subsequently applied to these data indicate that even in lesions with an apparently clear-cut cytokeratin profile, exceptions may occur with alarming frequency especially in units dealing with a large number of specimens where such exceptions occur several times each year. For example, almost all of ovarian cancers are CK 7-positive on Chu and Weiss's aggregate data but the confidence intervals are only 98.1–99.9% implying that up to one in fifty of these lesions are CK 7-negative.[30] When one examines the confidence intervals for ovarian cancer subtypes even greater inconsistencies can be expected (mucinous tumours have a CI of 90.1–98.8%, non-mucinous cancers a CI of 92.9–98.1%) so that up to one in ten of mucinous and one in twelve of non-mucinous lesions may not express this cytokeratin.

On the other hand, based on confidence intervals applied to Chen and Weiss's aggregate data, up to 16.6% (or one in six) of non-mucinous lesions may be CK 20-positive (mean 12.5%, CI 9.3–16.6%). Comparison of the results of a meta-analysis of cytokeratin expression in ovary and bowel in those series in which tumours at both sites were examined shows an odds ratio for CK 7 in the ovary versus colon of 103.56 but again there is a wide 95% confidence interval (41.62–257.69). The odds ratio for CK 20 expression in colon versus ovary is 43.52 (95% CI 20.65–91.72).

These results imply that in some cases at least the cytokeratin profile, if taken in isolation and examined on the assumption that ovarian cancer is always CK 7-positive and CK 20-negative, will be misleading. One would of course assume that this would not occur if the case were handled by an experienced pathologist.

There is a further complication when one examines the results from the individual studies which comprise the tables prepared by Chu and Weiss,[1] justified because of the variation of antibodies, incubation methods and systems for scoring the results employed where as few as 83% of cases of ovarian cancer might be expected to react to CK 7 and as many as 57% may react to CK 20. In contrast, up to 23% of colon cancers could be expected to react to CK 7 and only 70.9% react to CK 20.

## USE OF CYTOKERATINS IN CONFIRMING UNUSUAL DIAGNOSIS

Although tumours may occur typically at a particular site their overall incidence may be low and hence even a specialist pathologist may rarely encounter such an entity. In this situation, an appropriate immunoperoxidase reaction may re-assure the pathologist that the diagnosis is correct or prompt him or her to seek advice if unexpected reactions occur.

Merkel cell carcinomas are more likely to react to antibodies to CK 20 than are primary malignant melanomas or metastases from neuroendocrine carcinoma. The site of the antibody reaction within the cells may also be helpful. Merkel cell carcinoma was found to be reactive with antibodies to CK 20 (23/26 cases) and demonstrated at least focal perinuclear punctuate reaction pattern in 17 of them[31,32] with faint localised punctate staining in further case. Three of the CK 20-negative cases showed punctate staining with CAM 5.2. Punctate expression of cytokeratin detected with CAM 5.2 was found in small cell carcinoma of the bladder.[33] CK 7 expression may help in confirming a diagnosis of endometrioid adenocarcinoma of the ovary, particularly in differentiating between an endometrioid carcinoma with sex cord differentiation which morphologically may mimic a granulosa cell tumour.[34] Placed in context, an antibody panel that includes EMA and inhibin is of greater help.[35]

## ESTABLISHING COMMON DIAGNOSES WITH AN UNUSUAL MORPHOLOGY

The results of immunoperoxidase staining with cytokeratin antibodies may be misleading if examined in isolation. This is especially a problem if the antibody applied does not detect the cytokeratin profile likely to be expressed by the lesion suspected at that site. A case report by Gray et al.[36] highlights the importance of selecting an appropriate antibody panel to confirm the morphological diagnosis and exclude likely differential diagnoses. In this, a tumour that was essentially negative with AE 1/3 was diagnosed as an atypical fibroxanthoma. After it recurred, the case was reviewed and studied with a new antibody panel and it was found to be positive for 34 βE 12 resulting in a revised diagnosis of squamous cell carcinoma which was found, regrettably, to have lymph node metastases. Sigel et al.[37] found that 10 of 16 spindle cell squamous cell carcinomas were non-reactive for AE 1/3 but that 11 of 16 reacted for CK 5/6. Although AE 1/3 has a broad spectrum of reactivity, these antibodies (CK 5/6 and 34 βE 12) may be more helpful in the identification of squamous cell neoplasia.

Some series used antibody panels that included a single or restricted group of cytokeratin antibodies, each of which reacted to a broad spectrum of cytokeratins. In these instances, the presence of cytokeratin expression (as opposed to the examination of a cytokeratin profile) was found to be helpful in distinguishing extrarenal rhabdomyosarcoma tumour of soft tissue, sex cord stromal tumours (as opposed to carcinoma of ovary), myxoid transitional cell carcinoma of bladder (although some cross-over with other spindle cell bladder lesions was identified), lymphoepithelioma-like carcinoma of the cervix, pseudovascular squamous cell carcinoma of the cervix and malignant Sertoli cell tumour.

## USE OF ANTIBODY PANELS

It is difficult to conceive of a situation where a histopathologist when using immunohistochemical stains would not employ a panel of antibodies in diagnostic practice rather than one antibody in isolation. It is common in reported series and especially in case reports for panels of antibodies which include reagents to proteins other than cytokeratins to be used to refine diagnoses: these include studies of vasitis nodosa, urothelial polyp, pagetoid Bowen's disease, malignant Sertoli cell tumour, lymphoepithelioma-like carcinoma of the cervix, spindle cell squamous cell carcinoma of the skin, myxoid and sclerosing transitional cell carcinoma of the bladder, seminal vesicle carcinoma and pseudovascular squamous cell carcinoma of the cervix. Very few of these papers include control groups – the comparison of immune expression with that in tissues with diseases in the differential diagnosis on morphological grounds is often based on a literature review.

Although series have applied panels of antibodies to other diagnostic difficulties including distinguishing ovarian clear cell carcinoma from secretory endometrial carcinoma[3] and Merkel cell carcinoma from malignant melanoma, there is a dearth of literature comparing the relative value of antibodies to cytokeratins with those of other proteins. Where this has been attempted, the use of a combination of antibodies to different types of protein has been found to be beneficial in refining the diagnosis.[8] ( 1999). In the series of Lagendijk et al.,[8] some colonic tumours were CK 7- or Ca 125-positive and some ovarian cancers were CK 20- and CEA-positive. In practice, combinations of these antibodies may be applied to elucidating the origin of a disseminated intra-abdominal malignancy in as few as 10% of cases (local data).

## USES IN THE DIAGNOSIS OF SMALL VOLUME MALIGNANT DISEASE

One of the many challenging scenarios that the pathologist faces is identifying small volume disease at a metastatic site (the problem of small volume disease at a primary site of 'early invasion' usually being addressed by examining the continuity of basement membrane or basal or myoepithelial cell layer). Cytokeratin antibodies to detect metastatic tumour cells in inflammatory cutaneous metastases, lesions in the gut which may mimic solitary rectal ulcers and bone marrow (following tumour cell enrichment) have been described. The usefulness in detecting occult lymph node deposits in the breast was recently re-inforced[38] though the need to determine the clinical significance of these findings in terms of patient follow-up was highlighted. A negative reaction to cytokeratin antibodies may also be useful in proving that cells which might otherwise be confused with metastatic tumour cells in lymph node are not of epithelial origin (e.g. megakaryocytes are AE 1/3 negative).

Such findings in lymph nodes need to be interpreted with a full appreciation of the cytological morphology as non-metastatic cells such as fibroblastic reticulum cells react with anticytokeratin antibodies. Reactive mesothelial cells may occur in the subcapsular and medullary sinus of the lymph nodes of patients with effusions. These cells may react to cytokeratin antibodies but are negative to other cancer cell epithelial markers including CEA and EMA.

## CYTOKERATIN EXPRESSION IN CYTOLOGY SPECIMENS

Many cytopathology based studies of intermediate filament expression are still based on the use of one or two, usually broad-range, antibodies. Studies of the CK 19 protein concentration in benign and malignant pleural effusions measured by radioassay may stimulate further examination of cytokeratin profiles in cytological preparations.[39] A study of CK 8 and CK 17 expression in cervical smears has been advocated as the basis for an automated screening system.[40] As with histological specimens, CK 7 and CK 20 expression has been examined in fine needle aspirates and effusion specimens and was of diagnostic use provided that it was judiciously applied in the knowledge of the appropriate clinical history and morphological findings.

---

### Points of best practice

- The major use of antibodies to cytokeratins is in confirming a diagnosis made by an experienced pathologist rather than indicating a diagnosis to an inexperienced one.

- The evidence for the use of antibodies to cytokeratins to predict the likely site or sites of origin of metastatic tumours is sparse. Research to provide a justification for the practice is needed but should be easily achieved given the availability of microarrays..

- Although there is little evidence to support the view, when investigating the likely origin for a metastasis it would seem sensible to employ a panel that not only includes antibodies to cytokeratins but reagents to site and organ system specific markers such as CEA, Ca 125, PSA and antibodies to hormones which will confirm and possibly refine the diagnosis. Interpretation of the results of an antibody panel should not occur in isolation but on a background of a thorough clinical history, imaging results and morphological assessment.

## Points of best practice (continued)

- Primary tumours at the site of a presumed metastasis may express the same cytokeratin profile as the tumours that were likely to metastasise to this site.

- *In situ* and invasive neoplasia may be distinguished by identifying an intact myoepithelial layer in the former. In some conditions they may also be distinguished from each other or from reactive conditions by the demonstration of different cytokeratin profiles within the epithelial cells themselves.

- Cytokeratin profiles are proving to be of use in predicting the biological behaviour of lesions at some sites. This promising avenue of research requires more investigation.

- The use of cytokeratins in advancing the diagnosis of reactive lesions also warrants further investigation.

- To avoid misdiagnosis, when selecting a panel of antibodies to use in investigating a particular tumour the pathologist should be aware of the cytokeratin expression of the tumour cells, those of the tissues in the differential diagnoses, and the spectrum of cytokeratins to which the antibodies used react.

- The site of immunolocalization extracellularly within a tumour or in the cytoplasm of tumour cells rather than simply the presence or absence of a reaction may be important in making the differential diagnosis between some lesions.

- Even in situations, such as with the ovary and CK 7 and CK 20 expression, where most tumours might be expected to demonstrate a typical reaction profile, exceptions occur with sufficient frequency to be important in diagnosis. From the variation in the results in different series, pathologists will be aware that there are great differences in the frequency with which a reaction is recorded: it depends on the effects of different antibodies, methods of preparation, and scoring systems.

## ACKNOWLEDGEMENT

We are grateful to Miss Uzma Nazir in the preparation of this manuscript.

## References

1. Chu PG, Weiss LM. Keratin expression in human tissues and neoplasms. *Histopathology* 2002; **40**: 403–439.
2. Ronnett BM, Kurman RJ, Shmookler BM, Sugarbaker PH, Young RH. The morphologic spectrum of ovarian metastases of appendiceal adenocarcinomas. A clinicopathologic and immunohistochemical analysis of tumors often misinterpreted as primary ovarian tumors or metastatic tumors from other gastrointestinal sites. *Am J Surg Pathol* 1997; **21**: 1144–1155.
3. Young RH, Hart WR. Metastatic intestinal carcinomas simulating primary ovarian clear cell carcinoma and secretory endometrioid carcinoma. A clinicopathologic and immunohistochemical study of five cases. *Am J Surg Pathol* 1998; **22**: 805–815.

4. Yao DX, Hoda SA, Chiu A, Ying L, Rosen PP. Intraepidermal cytokeratin 7 immunoreactive cells in the non-neoplastic nipple may represent interepithelial extension of lactiferous duct cells. . *Histopathology* 2002; **40**: 230–236.

5. Tot T. Cytokeratins 20 and 7 as biomarkers; usefulness in discriminating primary from metastatic adenocarcinoma. *Eur J Cancer* 2002; **38**: 758–763.

6. Kummar S, Forarasi M, Canova A, Mota A, Cielielski T. Cytokeratin 7 and 20 staining for the diagnosis of lung and colorectal adenocarcinoma. *Br J Cancer* 2002; **86**: 1884–1887.

7. Loy TS, Calaluce RD, Keeney GL. Cytokeratin immunostaining in differentiating primary ovarian carcinoma from metastatic colonic adenocarcinoma. *Mod Pathol* 1996; **9**: 1040–1044.

8. Lagendijk JH, Mullink H, van Diest PJ, Meijer GA, Meijer CJLM. Immunohistochemical differentiation between primary adenocarcinomas of the ovary and ovarian metastases of colonic and breast origin. Comparison between a statistical and an intuitive approach. *J Clin Pathol* 1999; **52**: 283–290.

9. Rullier A, Le Bail B, Fawaz R, Blanc JF, Saric J, Biolulac-Sage P. Cytokeratin 7 and 20 expression in cholangiocarcinomas varies along the biliary tract but still differs from that in colorectal carcinoma metastasis. *Am J Surg Pathol* 2000; **24**: 870–876.

10. Chu PG, Weiss LM. Expression of cytokeratin 5/6 in epithelial neoplasms; an immunohistochemical study of 509 cases. *Mod Pathol* 2002; **15**: 6–9.

11. Carella R, Deleonardi G, D'Errico A *et al*. Immunohistochemical panels for differentiating epithelial malignant mesothelioma from lung adenocarcinoma. A study with logistic regression analysis. *Am J Surg Pathol* 2001; **25**: 43–50.

12. Attanoos RL, Webb R, Dojcinov SD, Gibbs AR. Value of mesothelial and epithelial antibodies in distinguishing diffuse peritoneal mesothelioma in females from serous papillary carcinoma of the ovary and peritoneum. *Histopathology* 2002; **40**: 237–244.

13. Chu PG, Lyda MH, Weiss LM. Cytokeratin 14 expression in epithelial neoplasms; a survey of 435 cases with emphasis on its value in differentiating squamous cell carcinomas from other epithelial tumours. *Histopathology* 2001; **39**: 9–16.

14. Heatley MK, Corke K. Involucrin and cytokeratin intermediate filament expression in cervical carcinoma. *Int J Gynaecol Cancer* 1998; **8**: 37–40.

15. Nolan LP, Heatley MK. The value of immunocytochemistry in distinguishing between clear cell carcinoma of the kidney and ovary. *Int J Gynecol Pathol* 2001; **20**: 155–159.

16. Joshi MG, Lee AK, Pedersen CA, Schnitt S, Camus MG, Hughes KS. The role of immunocytochemical markers in the differential diagnosis of proliferative and neoplastic lesions of the breast. *Mod Pathol* 1996; **9**: 57–62.

17. Heatley MK, Maxwell P, Whiteside C, Toner PG, Cytokeratin intermediate filament expression in benign and malignant breast epithelium. *J Clin Pathol* 1995; **48**: 26–32.

18. Abrahams NA, Ormsby AH, Brainard J. Validation of cytokeratin 5/6 as an effective substitute for keratin 903 in the differentiation of benign from malignant glands in prostate needle biopsies. *Histopathology* 2002; **41**: 35–41.

19. Hirokawa M, Carney A, Ohtsuki Y. Hyalinizing trabecular adenoma and papillary carcinoma of the thyroid gland express different cytokeratin patterns. *Am J Surg Pathol* 2000; **24**: 877–881.

20. Tsuji M, Kashihara T, Terada N, Mori H. An immunohistochemical study of hepatic atypical adenomatous hyperplasia, hepatocellular carcinoma, and cholangiocarcinoma with alpha-fetoprotein, carcinoembryonic antigen, CA19-9, epithelial membrane antigen, and cytokeratins 18 and 19. *Pathol Int* 1999; **49**: 310–317.

21. Sahoo S, Hoda SA, Rosai J, DeLellis RA. Cytokeratin 19 immunoreactivity in the diagnosis of papillary thyroid carcinoma: a note of caution. *Am J Clin Pathol* 2001; **116**: 696–702.

22. McKenney JK, Desai S, Cohen C, Amin MB. Discriminatory immunohistochemical staining of urothelial carcinoma *in situ* and non-neoplastic urothelium. `amm J Surg Pathol 2001; 25: 1074–8.

23. Harnden P, Mahmood N, Southgate J. Expression of cytokeratin 20 redefines urothelial papillomas of the bladder. *Lancet* 1999; **353**: 974–977.

24. Cheng L, Cheville JC, Sebo TJ, Eble JN, Bostwick DG. Atypical nephrogenic metaplasia of the urinary tract. A precursor lesion? *Cancer* 2000; **88**: 853–861.

25. Russo L, Woolnough E, Khan MS, Heatley MK. An immunohistochemical study of the rete ovarii and epoophoron. *Pathology* 2000; **32**: 77–83.

26. Ormsby AH, Goldblum J, Rice TW, Richter JE, Falk GW, Vaezi MF. Cytokeratin subsets can reliably distinguish Barrett's esophagus from intestinal metaplasia of the stomach. *Hum Pathol* 1998; **30**: 288–294.

27. Goldstein NS, Soman A, Gordon SC. Portal tract eosinophils and hepatocyte cytokeratin 7 immunoreactivity helps distinguish early-stage, mildly active primary biliary cirrhosis and autoimmune hepatitis. *Am J Clin Pathol* 2001; **116**: 846–853.

28. Lehr H-A, Folpe A, Yaziji H, Kommoss F, Gown AM. Cytokeratin 8 immunostaining pattern and E-cadherin expression distinguish lobular from ductal breast carcinoma. *Am J Clin Pathol* 2000; **114**: 190–196.

29. Liberman E, Weidner N. Papillary and follicular neoplasms of the thyroid gland. Differential immunohistochemical staining with high molecular weight keratin and involucrin. *Appl Immunohistochem Mol Morphol* 2000; **8**: 42–48.

30. Heatley MK. Keratin expression in human tissues and neoplasms. *Histopathology* 2002; **41**: 365–366.

31. Nicholson SA, McDermott MB, Swanson PE, Wick MR. CD99 and cytokeratin 20 in small cell and basaloid tumors of the skin. *Appl Immunohistochem Mol Morphol* 2000; **8**: 37–41.

32. Jensen K, Kohler S, Rouse RV. Cytokeratin staining in Merkel cell carcinoma: an immunohistochemical study of cytokeratins 5/6, 7, 17 and 20. *Appl Immunohistochem Mol Morphol* 2000; **8**: 310–315.

33. Iczkowski KA, Shanks JH, Allsbrook WC *et al*. Small cell carcinoma of urinary bladder is differentiated from urothelial carcinoma by chromogranin expression, absence of CD44 variant 6 expression, a unique pattern of cytokeratin expression, and more intense gamma-enolase expression. *Histopathology* 1999; **35**: 150–156.

34. Guerrieri C, Franlund B, Malmstrom H, Boeryd B. Ovarian endometrioid carcinomas simulating sex cord-stromal tumors: a study using inhibin and cytokeratin 7. *Int J Gynecol Pathol* 1998; **17**: 266–271.

35. Ripel MA, Perlman EJ Seidman JD, Kurman RJ, Sherman ME. Inhibin and epithelial membrane antigen immunohistochemistry assist in the diagnosis of sex cord-stromal tumors and provide clues to the histogenesis of hypercalcemic small cell carcinomas. *Int J Gynecol Pathol* 1998; **17**: 46–53.

36. Gray Y, Robidoux HJ, Farrell DS, Robinson-Bostom L. Squamous cell carcinoma detected by high-molecular-weight cytokeratin immunostaining mimicking atypical fibroxanthoma. *Arch Pathol Lab Med* 2001; **125**: 799–802.

37. Sigel JE, Skacel M, Bergfeld WF, House NS, Rabkin MS, Goldblum JR. The utility of cytokeratin 5/6 in the recognition of cutaneous spindle cell squamous cell carcinoma. *J Cutan Pathol* 2001; **28**: 520–524.

38. Freneaux P, Nos C, Salamon A-V *et al*. Histological detection of minimal metastatic involvement in axillary sentinel nodes: a rational basis for a sensitive methodology usable in daily practice. *Mod Pathol* 2002; **15**: 641–646.

39. Lee YC, Knox BS, Garrett JE. Use of cytokeratin fragments 19.1 and 19.21 (Cyfra 21-1) in the differentiation of malignant and benign pleural effusions. *Aust NZ J Med* 1999; **29**: 765–769.

40. Martens J, Baars J, Smedts F *et al*. Can keratin 8 and 17 immunohistochemistry be of diagnostic value in cervical cytology? A feasibility study. *Cancer* 1999; **87**: 87–92.

W.G. McCluggage

3

# Metaplasias in the female genital tract

Metaplasia is defined as 'the abnormal transformation of an adult, fully differentiated tissue of one kind into a differentiated tissue of another kind'.[1] Perhaps the best known examples are squamous metaplasia of the cervix and of the pseudostratified columnar ciliated epithelium of the bronchial and tracheal mucosa of cigarette smokers. Epithelial metaplasia occurs in many organs. Connective tissue metaplasia, such as the formation of metaplastic bone, cartilage and adipose tissue from other connective tissues also occurs. This chapter reviews metaplasia in the female genital system, organs which are amongst the most commonly involved by metaplastic processes.

## METAPLASIAS IN THE FEMALE GENITAL SYSTEM

The Müllerian-derived epithelium which lines most of the female genital system is well known for its capacity to differentiate into epithelium of ciliated, mucinous, endometrioid, transitional and squamous types.[2] The abdominal and pelvic peritoneum, part of the secondary Müllerian system, can also undergo metaplasia into the various Müllerian epithelia. Conditions such as endosalpingiosis and endocervicosis are regarded as examples of Müllerian metaplasia. and will be described briefly. This review will concentrate on metaplasia of the uterine corpus and cervix as these are the most common sites of metaplasia and result in the most diagnostic difficulty. Metaplasia occasionally occurs in other parts of the female genital system, such as mucinous and transitional metaplasia involving the mucosa of the fallopian tube.

**Dr W.G. McCluggage** FRCPath
Consultant Pathologist, Department of Pathology, Royal Group of Hospitals Trust, Grosvenor Road, Belfast BT12 6BL, Northern Ireland, UK
Tel: +44 2890 240503 Ext 2563; Fax: +44 2890 233643; E-mail: glenn.mccluggage@bll.n-i.nhs.uk

**Table 1** International Society of Gynecological Pathologists' classification of endometrial epithelial metaplasias

Squamous metaplasia and morules
Mucinous metaplasia (including intestinal)
Ciliary change
Hobnail cell change
Clear cell change
Eosinophilic cell change (including oncocytic)
Surface syncytial change
Papillary proliferation
Arias-Stella change

## ENDOMETRIAL EPITHELIAL METAPLASIA

The normal endometrial epithelium is composed of cuboidal to columnar cells with faintly eosinophilic cytoplasm. Ciliated cells are common, especially in the proliferative phase; their presence should not be taken as indicative of tubal or ciliated metaplasia. The International Society of Gynecological Pathologists' classification of endometrial epithelial metaplasia is given in Table 1. These commonly co-exist with one another. Endometrial epithelial metaplasia is a group of non-neoplastic lesions (metaplasia often co-exists with endometrial hyperplasia or adenocarcinoma) in which the normal endometrial epithelium is replaced, focally or diffusely, by a different type of differentiated epithelium. Metaplasia is usually of non-secretory endometrium and may occur within polyps. Epithelial metaplasia is especially likely to occur in tamoxifen-associated endometrial polyps[3,4] and in non-polypoid endometrium and adenomyosis associated with tamoxifen usage.[5]

Epithelial metaplasia often co-exists with endometrial hyperplasia or carcinoma and should not be misdiagnosed as a malignant or pre-malignant lesion. Conversely, there is a risk of underdiagnosis of malignancy: mucinous adenocarcinomas of the endometrium may appear extremely bland and, especially in biopsy specimens, be mistaken for a non-neoplastic metaplastic process.[6–8]

It has been suggested that metaplasia is an inappropriate term for some of the lesions listed in Table 1 as it refers to the replacement of one type of epithelium by another that is inappropriate to that site. For this reason, some authors used the term 'change' rather than metaplasia. In this review, the terms 'metaplasia' and 'change' will be regarded as synonymous. Perhaps the best definition of endometrial epithelial metaplasia was that proffered by Hendrickson and Kempson in 1980.[9] Endometrial epithelial metaplasia was defined as the replacement of the normal glandular epithelium by cells that are either not encountered in the normal epithelium or, if present, are usually inconspicuous.[9] The classification of endometrial metaplasias proposed by Hendrickson and Kempson forms the basis for the International Society of Gynecological Pathologists' classification.

## CLINICAL ASSOCIATIONS

Endometrial epithelial metaplasia can co-exist with endometrial hyperplasia or carcinoma.[10,11] Most examples of metaplasia are found in postmenopausal women.[9] Often, there is an association with exogenous hormone therapy, especially unopposed oestrogens. Other aetiological factors are an intra-uterine device, chronic endometritis, and pyometra; the latter two conditions are especially associated with squamous metaplasia. Endometrial epithelial metaplasia also occurs in polypoid and non-polypoid endometrium of patients taking tamoxifen.[3,4] Metaplasia by itself is not associated with clinical symptoms but if there is associated endometrial hyperplasia or carcinoma there may be symptoms related to these.

## SQUAMOUS METAPLASIA WITH MORULES

Squamous metaplasia is the commonest form of metaplasia in the endometrium.[9] Although this may be a focal finding, it may be widespread and involve most of the endometrium. Microscopically, it is composed of bland squamous cells with eosinophilic cytoplasm (Fig. 1). Central necrosis may be present and has no sinister connotation. Squamous metaplasia is common in endometrioid adenocarcinoma[12] and in endometrial hyperplasia: these conditions should be excluded by careful examination of the glandular elements. The squamous component in endometrioid adenocarcinoma may be morphologically benign, malignant or indeterminate and have a variety of morphological patterns.[13] The World Health Organization (WHO) categorises adenocarcinoma with squamous differentiation as a variant of endometrioid adenocarcinoma and no longer accepts terms such as adenoacanthoma and adenosquamous carcinoma.

Morules differ from mature squamous metaplasia in that they lack keratinisation and intercellular bridges. Morules and foci of mature squamous metaplasia often co-exist. An endometrial lesion in which squamous elements, usually in the form of morules, are extremely common and prominent is an atypical polypoid adenomyoma.[14–16] This usually arises in the lower uterine segment and is composed of architecturally complex endometrial glands which often have cytological atypia intermingled with bundles of smooth

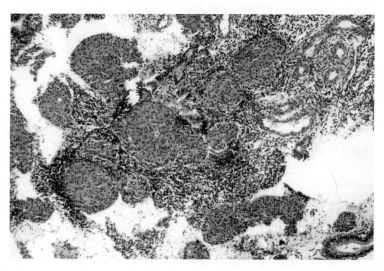

**Fig. 1** Metaplastic squamous epithelium in the form of morules within endometrium.

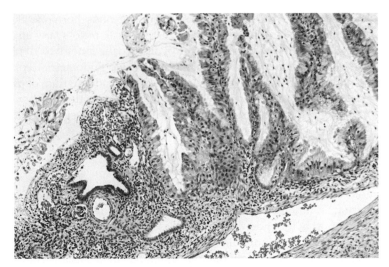

**Fig. 2** Mucinous metaplasia with complex architecture within endometrium. In such instances a well-differentiated mucinous adenocarcinoma may be considered.

muscle. This can mimic well-differentiated invasive endometrial adenocarcinoma. Extensive squamous metaplasia of the endometrium also occurs in association with pyometra, endometritis, cervical stenosis or an intra-uterine device. Endometrial squamous metaplasia occurs secondary to progestogen therapy.[17]

## MUCINOUS METAPLASIA

This is a rarer form of endometrial metaplasia:[9,18] the diagnosis should be reserved for cases in which the endometrial epithelial cells are replaced by cells with abundant mucin-containing cytoplasm (Fig. 2), which resemble endocervical cells. Normal endometrial epithelial cells contain some intracytoplasmic mucin, especially with a luminal distribution, and so abundant mucin is required for the diagnosis. Rarely, intestinal metaplasia has been described in the endometrium, in which the mucinous epithelium contains goblet cells.[19] Enteric type mucins may be demonstrable without morphological evidence of intestinal metaplasia.[20] This is also the case in the cervix.[21]

As with other types of endometrial metaplasia, mucinous metaplasia can co-exist with endometrial hyperplasia. An important diagnostic consideration is that mucinous adenocarcinoma of the endometrium can be cytologically bland.[6–8] As mucinous metaplasia of the endometrium can have a complex growth pattern, it can be difficult to distinguish between mucinous metaplasia and well-differentiated adenocarcinoma, especially in endometrial biopsy tissue. Nucci *et al.*[22] divided mucinous proliferations of the endometrium into three categories depending on the degree of architectural complexity. With any architecturally complex mucinous proliferation in the endometrium, the diagnosis of well-differentiated mucinous adenocarcinoma should be considered. Well-differentiated mucinous adenocarcinomas of the endometrium with a microglandular growth pattern can also have a close morphological resemblance to cervical microglandular hyperplasia.[6–8] There

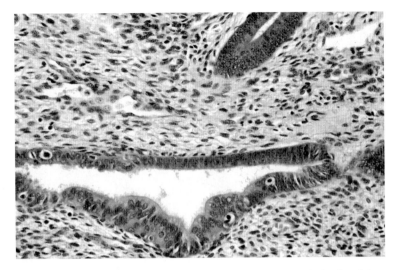

**Fig. 3** Ciliated metaplasia within endometrium. Most of the epithelial cells of the lower gland contain cilia on the luminal aspect.

may be a severe neutrophilic infiltrate in both. In biopsy tissue, a diagnosis of mucinous adenocarcinoma should be considered in a lesion resembling cervical microglandular hyperplasia in a postmenopausal patient, although cervical microglandular hyperplasia rarely occurs in this age group. A microglandular growth pattern is especially likely to be found on the surface of endometrial adenocarcinoma.[23] Vimentin staining may be of use: adenocarcinoma usually stains positively and microglandular hyperplasia is negative.[24] Rarely, mucinous metaplasia in the endometrium is accompanied by mucinous lesions elsewhere in the female genital system.[25]

## CILIATED OR TUBAL METAPLASIA

Ciliated endometrial epithelial cells are a normal phenomenon, so a diagnosis of ciliated metaplasia (Fig. 3) should be made only when one or more endometrial glands are lined predominantly by ciliated cells.[9] Ciliated cells often have very eosinophilic cytoplasm. As with other types of epithelial metaplasia, ciliated cells are found in non-neoplastic and hyperplastic endometrium. The presence or absence of hyperplasia is evaluated by the usual variables. Isolated ciliated cells are commonly found in endometrial adenocarcinoma and a 'ciliated adenocarcinoma' has been described.[26] This is a variant of endometrioid adenocarcinoma in which the tumour is composed predominantly of ciliated cells. This variant is recognised in the WHO classification of endometrial carcinoma.

## CLEAR CELL METAPLASIA

Clear cell metaplasia is characterised by replacement of endometrial epithelial cells by cells with abundant clear cytoplasm (Fig. 4).[9] This may be found in the endometrium in pregnancy. Especially when florid, clear cell metaplasia may

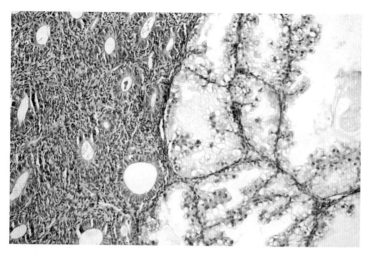

**Fig. 4** Clear cell metaplasia within endometrium. In this case a diagnosis of clear cell carcinoma was considered but the subsequent hysterectomy contained no tumour.

be misdiagnosed as clear cell carcinoma. Distinction is based on the bland nuclear features and the fact that in clear cell metaplasia the endometrial glands are of normal architecture and distribution. When clear cell metaplasia involves architecturally complex glands, the distinction from clear cell carcinoma may be very difficult, especially as clear cell carcinoma may be cytologically bland. Other features favouring clear cell metaplasia over clear cell carcinoma include focality of the lesion, absence of a visible tumour on hysteroscopy, absence of stromal invasion and presence of oestrogen receptor positivity. Most ovarian clear cell carcinomas are oestrogen receptor negative.

## HOBNAIL CELL METAPLASIA

Hobnail cell metaplasia is characterised by the presence of cells with rounded apical blebs.[9] Hobnail cell metaplasia is usually a reparative phenomenon after endometrial biopsy. It also occurs in pregnancy. Hobnail cells are also characteristic of clear cell carcinoma and this may enter into the differential diagnosis, especially if there is accompanying clear cell metaplasia. Criteria useful in the distinction of hobnail cell metaplasia from clear cell carcinoma are similar to those used in distinction of the latter from clear cell metaplasia.

## EOSINOPHILIC (OXYPHIL, ONCOCYTIC) METAPLASIA

Eosinophilic metaplasia is characterised by the presence of epithelial cells with abundant eosinophilic cytoplasm (Fig. 5).[9] The cytoplasm may be granular, in which case the term oncocytic metaplasia has been used.[27] Ultrastructurally, abundant cytoplasmic mitochondria may be present as is characteristic of oncocytes in other organs.[27] Some degree of cytoplasmic eosinophilia is commonly found in endometrial epithelial cells and does not alone warrant a diagnosis of eosinophilic metaplasia.

The main differential diagnosis, especially when there is architectural complexity, is the eosinophilic or oxyphilic variant of endometrioid

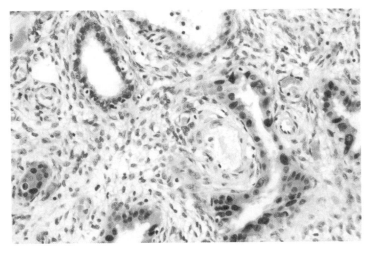

**Fig. 5** Eosinophilic (oncocytic) metaplasia within endometrium. There is a degree of nuclear atypia.

adenocarcinoma.[27,28] The cells in eosinophilic metaplasia can have a worrying degree of nuclear atypia (Fig. 5), similar to the degenerative nuclear atypia that can involve oncocytic cells in other organs. Distinction from adenocarcinoma is made on the absence of a visible lesion on hysteroscopy, absence of severe cytological atypia, and absence of stromal invasion.

## PAPILLARY SYNCYTIAL METAPLASIA

Papillary syncytial metaplasia in most cases represents a reparative phenomenon after menstrual shedding or recent endometrial sampling (Fig. 6)[9,29]. It is one of the commoner forms of endometrial metaplasia. Histologically it is characterised by a syncytium of endometrial epithelial cells which have small glandular lumina and papillae which lack fibrovascular

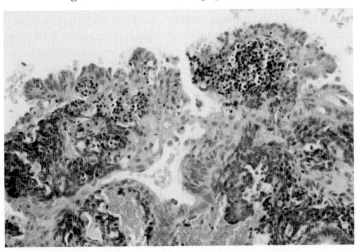

**Fig. 6** Papillary syncytial metaplasia within endometrium. Note that this is associated with stromal breakdown.

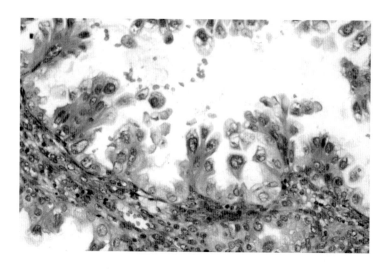

**Fig. 7** Arias-Stella reaction within endometrium. Note the nuclear enlargement and atypia.

stromal cores. The cells usually have eosinophilic cytoplasm and there is often a heavy neutrophil infiltrate. There may be mild nuclear atypia and degenerative nuclear features are common.

An important consideration is that foci similar to papillary syncytial metaplasia (and to cervical microglandular hyperplasia) may occur on the surface of some endometrial adenocarcinomas.[23] The most important differential diagnosis of papillary syncytial metaplasia is papillary adenocarcinoma of endometrioid or serous type. The changes of papillary syncytial metaplasia are limited to the surface and are often associated with signs of breakdown.

A lesion recently described in detail by Lehman and Hart[30] which is most frequently seen in endometrial polyps is characterised by papillary proliferations with fibrovascular cores. The epithelial cells are bland or have mild nuclear atypia. Other metaplastic changes may accompany this. This lesion is mentioned here because, like papillary syncytial metaplasia, it has a papillary appearance and so could be misdiagnosed as papillary endometrial carcinoma.

## ARIAS-STELLA CHANGE

The Arias-Stella change is almost always seen in pregnancy or trophoblastic disease, and occasionally with hormone therapy:[31] rarely, there is no association.[32] Histologically, there may be cellular stratification, secretory activity and enlargement of the epithelial cell nuclei and cytoplasm (Fig. 7). Nuclei show considerable atypia and occasional mitotic figures may be present. Atypical mitoses have been found.[33] Recently five histological variants have been described: minimally atypical, early secretory pattern, hypersecretory pattern, regenerative (proliferative or non-secretory) pattern, and monstrous cell pattern.[34] The most important differential diagnosis is clear cell carcinoma but the diagnosis of Arias-Stella change is usually straightforward if there is a history of pregnancy or if other morphological features of pregnancy are present. In addition, the Arias-Stella change involves pre-existing endometrial glands and there is no evidence of stromal infiltration.

## ENDOMETRIAL MESENCHYMAL METAPLASIA

Mesenchymal metaplasia may involve the endometrial stroma. This form of metaplasia is rare.

### SMOOTH MUSCLE METAPLASIA

This is the most common mesenchymal metaplasia in the endometrium. It is thought that a multipotential cell exists in the uterus which has the capacity to differentiate into endometrial stroma and smooth muscle.[35] This is in keeping with the observation that there is immunohistochemical overlap between endometrial stromal and smooth muscle neoplasms[36,37] and that hybrid endometrial stromal-smooth muscle neoplasms exist.[38] It is common to find small foci of typical smooth muscle in the endometrial stroma (Fig. 8). Some authors have referred to these as intra-endometrial leiomyomas. It is possible that some of these foci are artifactual, the result of the irregular nature of the normal endometrial–myometrial junction but others undoubtedly reflect the capacity of endometrial stroma to differentiate into smooth muscle.

### CARTILAGINOUS AND OSSEOUS METAPLASIA

Rarely, foci of bone or cartilage are found within the endometrium.[39–41] In many cases, it is likely that these are of fetal origin. This is especially likely to be the case if these tissues are found in the endometrium of a young woman with a past history of abortion. In other cases, the cartilage or bone is truly metaplastic. This may be seen in normal endometrium but perhaps more commonly occurs in the stroma of an endometrial neoplasm.[42] Benign osseous or cartilaginous metaplasia in an endometrial carcinoma should not be mistaken for the sarcomatous component of a carcinosarcoma.

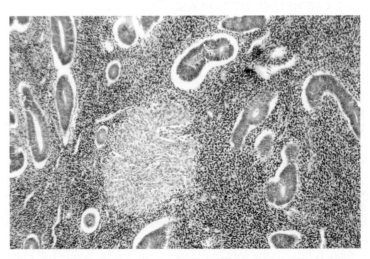

**Fig. 8** Well circumscribed collection of smooth muscle fibres within endometrial stroma.

## GLIAL METAPLASIA

In most cases, glial tissue (confirmed if necessary by positive immuno-histochemical staining with GFAP) in the endometrium is presumed to be a consequence of a previous abortion.[43,44] Histological support for this may come from the identification of other elements such as cartilage or bone. Glial tissue in the endometrium is rare and the chief differential diagnostic consideration is a teratoma.

## ADIPOSE METAPLASIA

Small metaplastic foci of adipose tissue may be found in endometrial stroma.[45] Adipose tissue may also rarely be seen in the stroma of an endometrial polyp. If found in an endometrial biopsy or curettage specimen, the possibility of uterine perforation must be raised. Other explanations for the presence of fat in endometrial biopsies include lipoma, lipoleiomyoma, rare uterine hamartomatous-like lesions containing fat[46] and adipose tissue as a component of a uterine carcinosarcoma.

## EXTRAMEDULLARY HAEMATOPOIESIS

Extramedullary haematopoiesis, recognised by the presence of megakaryo-cytes, erythroid and myeloid precursors, is occasionally seen in the endometrium.[47–49] As with several of the mesenchymal metaplasias described above, these elements may be fetal in origin as a consequence of a previous abortion. In other cases there is no such history but rather an association with an underlying haematological disorder. If extramedullary haematopoiesis is identified in the endometrium in the absence of other tissues, an underlying haematological disorder should be considered and investigated. In some cases, extramedullary haematopoiesis appears to be an incidental finding of no clinical significance.

## CERVICAL EPITHELIAL METAPLASIA

In late fetal life, the cervical canal is lined by columnar epithelium and the ectocervix by non-keratinised stratified squamous epithelium. The junction between the two is known as the original squamocolumnar junction. Later the columnar epithelium close to the original squamocolumnar junction undergoes metaplastic change into squamous epithelium. This area is known as the transformation zone of the cervix and persists into adult life. The extent of metaplastic change varies throughout a woman's reproductive life in response to hormonal changes and other influences.

Squamous metaplasia occurring in the transformation zone of the cervix begins as a patchy process, the foci of squamous metaplasia enlarging and eventually fusing. The metaplasia involves both the surface epithelium and underlying crypts. Squamous metaplasia is extremely common in the cervix and should be seen as a normal phenomenon rather than an abnormal pathological process. Especially when the metaplastic squamous epithelium is mature, there is little in the way of diagnostic difficulty. Before full maturation

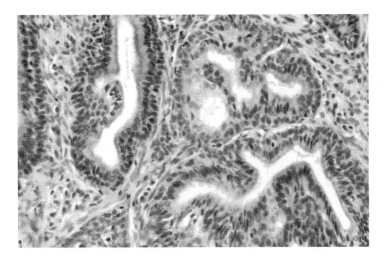

**Fig. 9** Reserve cell hyperplasia involving endocervical glands.

is reached, though, there are stages of reserve cell hyperplasia and immature squamous metaplasia, both of which may cause diagnostic difficulty.

## RESERVE CELL HYPERPLASIA

This is the first stage in the metaplastic process which eventually results in the transformation of columnar epithelium into mature squamous epithelium. Reserve cell hyperplasia is characterised by the presence of a layer of cuboidal or low columnar cells with clear cytoplasm situated immediately beneath the normal endocervical cells but separated from the stroma by a basement membrane (Fig. 9). This results in a histological double cell layer. Reserve cells are normally present in the columnar epithelium of the cervix but are usually inconspicuous. Occasionally the presence of a double cell layer may be confusing and result in consideration of cervical glandular intra-epithelial neoplasia (CGIN). However, the histological appearances are characteristic and CGIN can be excluded if attention is paid to the nuclear details. Eventually, reserve cells acquire more abundant eosinophilic cytoplasm during the process of transformation into squamous cells.

## IMMATURE AND MATURE SQUAMOUS METAPLASIA

The progression of reserve cell hyperplasia results in the development of a multilayered epithelium with features of both squamous and glandular differentiation. Squamous features are usually most prominent near the base of the epithelium while towards the surface, glandular differentiation is apparent in the form of cytoplasmic mucin (Fig. 10). Eventually, the columnar epithelium is completely replaced by immature squamous epithelium. This differs from mature squamous epithelium by lack of surface maturation and less intra-cytoplasmic glycogen. There is often a sharp demarcation from adjacent mature squamous epithelium. As the process continues, the immature metaplastic squamous epithelium is converted to mature squamous epithelium.

39

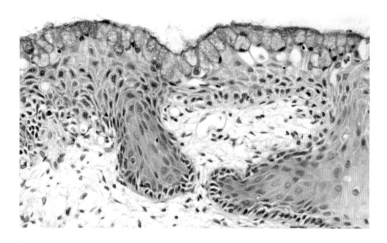

**Fig. 10** Immature squamous metaplasia. A layer of mucin-containing cells is still present on the surface

Histologically, this is recognised by the presence of endocervical crypts deep to mature squamous epithelium (crypts are not found deep to native mature squamous epithelium).

Immature squamous metaplasia may be mistaken for cervical intra-epithelial neoplasia (CIN) and the term 'atypical immature squamous metaplasia' has been used for cases with nuclear atypia.[50,51] Immature squamous metaplasia is distinguished from CIN by the presence of a uniform population of cells with scant cytoplasm and nuclei which lack significant pleomorphism. The nuclei are not hyperchromatic and, though mitotic figures may be present, abnormal mitoses are not seen. The presence on the surface of cells containing mucin may also be useful in distinguishing immature squamous metaplasia from CIN. I think that the term atypical immature squamous metaplasia is best avoided as a diagnosis because it creates a problem for the gynaecologist – there are no clear guidelines for the management of this lesion and reproducibility of this diagnosis among histopathologists is likely to be poor. A minor degree of nuclear atypia is acceptable in immature squamous metaplasia. It should be remembered that CIN commonly involves immature metaplastic squamous epithelium. In this instance, grading of the CIN may be difficult. In my opinion, rather than using the term atypical immature squamous metaplasia, a diagnosis of CIN should be made when there is significant nuclear atypia involving immature metaplastic squamous epithelium. When grading of CIN is difficult, a diagnosis of CIN unclassified should be made with a statement on whether this is likely to be low grade (CIN 1) or high grade (CIN 2–3).

Koilocytosis may also involve immature metaplastic squamous epithelium and result in atypical epithelial changes. Studies of cases of atypical immature squamous metaplasia, using HPV typing with careful follow-up, have shown that some cases of atypical immature squamous metaplasia are probably a variant of high-grade CIN.[50] This further underlines the necessity to distinguish the cases of atypical immature squamous metaplasia which represent true CIN. It is likely that cases diagnosed as atypical immature squamous metaplasia are a heterogenous group of lesions that includes

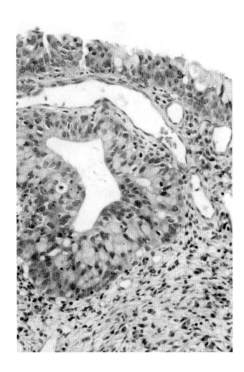

**Fig. 11** Stratified mucinous intra-epithelial lesion involving surface epithelium and underlying endocervical gland.

dysplastic and non-dysplastic lesions. Every effort should be made to separate these lesions histologically and the term atypical immature squamous metaplasia as a diagnosis is best avoided.

Another lesion which deserves mention because of its potential confusion with immature squamous metaplasia is the stratified mucinous intra-epithelial lesion characterised by Park and colleagues.[52] This lesion involves the surface epithelium and underlying endocervical crypts and is characterised by a multilayered epithelium resembling CIN (Fig. 11). However, in addition many cytoplasmic mucin droplets are present throughout the full thickness of the epithelium, resulting in an appearance reminiscent of atypical immature squamous metaplasia. Stratified mucinous intra-epithelial lesion is associated with more extreme nuclear pleomorphism and hyperchromasia and a higher proliferation index, demonstrable by MIB1 staining, than immature squamous metaplasia. In stratified mucinous intra-epithelial lesion, cytoplasmic mucin droplets are present throughout the full epithelial thickness whereas with immature squamous metaplasia they are located close to the surface. In addition, stratified mucinous intra-epithelial lesion is almost always associated with CIN or CGIN and commonly with an invasive carcinoma which may be squamous, glandular or adenosquamous in type. It has been considered that stratified mucinous intra-epithelial lesion is a form of reserve cell neoplasia and a marker of phenotypic instability.[52] When this lesion is identified on a small cervical biopsy, the possibility of co-existent CIN, CGIN or invasive carcinoma should be considered.

## TRANSITIONAL METAPLASIA

Transitional cell metaplasia of the cervix is uncommon and is usually an incidental finding in postmenopausal women.[53,54] There is usually no apparent

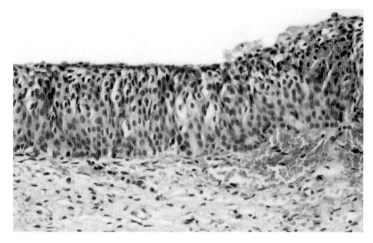

**Fig. 12** Transitional cell metaplasia involving cervix.

cause though transitional cell metaplasia has been described in the cervices of transsexual women receiving androgen therapy, suggesting that hormonal factors such as hypo-oestrogenism may be implicated in the pathogenesis.[55] Occasionally, presentation is with an abnormal cervical smear and transitional cell metaplasia may be recognised on cytological preparations.[56] Transitional cell metaplasia may involve both the surface epithelium and underlying endocervical glands and is more common on the ectocervix. Histologically, it is characterised by cells with pale, uniform, ovoid to spindle-shaped nuclei which may contain grooves (Fig. 12). A useful diagnostic feature, not always present, is that in the deeper layers of the epithelium the nuclei are usually orientated at right angles to the basement membrane whereas superficially they are parallel to it. A superficial layer of umbrella cells may be present in some cases. Mitotic figures are rare or absent. The main problem in diagnosis is the superficial resemblance to CIN 3, especially in those cases with tightly packed nuclei and a low nuclear-to-cytoplasmic ratio. The bland nuclear features, lack of mitotic figures, presence of nuclear grooves and different architectural arrangement of cells in the deep and superficial layers of epithelium indicate the correct diagnosis. Occasionally, dysplastic change may involve transitional cell metaplasia creating obvious diagnostic difficulties.

Transitional cell metaplasia of the cervix has been shown immuno-histochemically to express some markers of urothelial differentiation but not to exhibit a complete urothelial phenotype:[57] CK 20 and asymmetric unit membrane, markers associated with full differentiation in urothelium, are not expressed in cervical transitional cell metaplasia.[57]

## TUBAL METAPLASIA, TUBO-ENDOMETRIAL METAPLASIA AND ENDOMETRIOSIS

Tubal and tubo-endometrial metaplasia are very common in the cervix.[58,59] In some cases the epithelium has predominantly tubal differentiation with abundant cilia (Fig. 13) while in other cases there is a more endometrioid appearance with non-ciliated cuboidal and columnar epithelial cells.

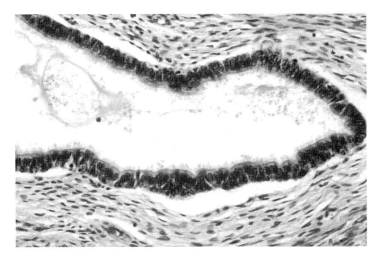

**Fig. 13** Tubo-endometrial metaplasia involving endocervical glands. Note the presence of cilia.

Endometrial stroma may also be present. In cases with endometrial epithelium and stroma, a diagnosis of endometriosis is justified.[60] It should be remembered that there are two main types of cervical endometriosis. Superficial endometriosis occurs superficially in the cervix and there is usually no association with pelvic endometriosis.[60] Although some cases may be due to implantation of endometrial tissue, other cases, especially when associated with tubal differentiation, are probably the result of a metaplastic process similar to tubo-endometrial metaplasia. Deep cervical endometriosis, on the other hand, occurs deep within the cervical stroma towards the external surface and is often associated with pelvic endometriosis. Glands lined by ciliated epithelium are a normal finding high up the endocervical canal close to the isthmus. When tubo-endometrial metaplasia occurs in the region of the transformation zone of the cervix, especially when florid, it is often a reparative phenomenon secondary to a previous procedure such as loop or cone biopsy. However, in many cases there is no such history. Both tubo-endometrial metaplasia and superficial endometriosis can have nuclear atypia and mitotic figures may be present, resulting in consideration of CGIN. When there is significant atypia this has been referred to as atypical tubo-endometrial metaplasia. In addition, especially in cases where there has been prior surgery to the cervix with stromal fibrosis, the features may suggest a desmoplastic stromal reaction.[61] Crypts involved by tubo-endometrial metaplasia may also be situated deep in the cervical stroma and may line deep Nabothian cysts. These features can rarely result in consideration of invasive adenocarcinoma. In cases of superficial endometriosis where there has been previous haemorrhage, the stroma may become fibrotic also resulting in consideration of a desmoplastic stromal reaction.

The presence of cilia is always a useful pointer towards a non-neoplastic lesion but recently a ciliated variant of CGIN has been described (designated adenocarcinoma *in situ* of tubal type).[62] These cases were associated with typical and atypical tubal metaplasia and with tubal morphology, in the form

**Table 2** Characteristic staining patterns of tubo-endometrial metaplasia, endometriosis, microglandular hyperplasia and high grade CGIN

|  | MIB1 | bcl-2 | p16 |
| --- | --- | --- | --- |
| Tubo-endometrial metaplasia | Negative or low | Diffuse | Negative or focal |
| Endometriosis | Negative or low | Diffuse | Negative or focal |
| Microglandular hyperplasia | Negative or low | Negative | Negative |
| High-grade CGIN | Intermediate or high | Negative | Diffuse |

of cilia, in the areas of CGIN. Ciliated CGIN undoubtedly exists but it is rare and most cases with atypia probably represent atypical tubo-endometrial metaplasia which has no malignant potential.

A panel of immunohistochemical stains comprising MIB1, bcl2 and p16 may be of value in the distinction of high grade CGIN from cervical tubo-endometrial metaplasia and endometriosis (and microglandular hyperplasia).[63] Characteristic staining patterns with each of the three antibodies are shown in Table 2. In general, high-grade CGIN has a high proliferation index with MIB1,[64] is negative with bcl2 and is diffusely positive with p16. Tubo-endometrial metaplasia and endometriosis usually have a low proliferation index with MIB1 (in occasional cases the MIB1 index is 30–50%); positivity with p16 is common though focal, unlike the diffuse staining of all cells which is characteristic of high-grade CGIN. Both tubo-endometrial metaplasia and endometriosis have constant diffuse cytoplasmic staining with bcl2.[65,66] Low-grade CGIN is not well characterised. In most cases of tubo-endometrial metaplasia and endometriosis, immuno-histochemistry is unnecessary and should always be carefully interpreted in the context of the morphological features.

## CERVICAL MICROGLANDULAR HYPERPLASIA

Microglandular hyperplasia is common within the cervix and is usually associated with exogenous hormone use or pregnancy.[67] It usually occurs in the reproductive age group. Although not a metaplasia, it is best categorised with these. Occasionally on colposcopic examination or direct visualisation of the cervix, a polypoid mass is seen but usually microglandular hyperplasia is an incidental microscopic finding. Histologically microglandular hyperplasia is characterised by closely packed glands, most of which are small but some of which may be cystically dilated (Fig. 14). Neutrophils and chronic inflammatory cells, especially plasma cells, are a characteristic feature. Crypts are lined with cuboidal or low columnar cells which commonly have subnuclear and supranuclear vacuolation. Reserve cell hyperplasia and immature squamous metaplasia often co-exist.

Most cases are typical and easily recognised as microglandular hyperplasia. Atypical features include the presence of marked stromal hyalinisation, oedema or myxoid change, signet-ring or spindle-shaped cells, solid or trabecular areas, and some degree of nuclear pleomorphism.[68] A correct diagnosis is facilitated by the presence of areas of typical microglandular hyperplasia, the knowledge that these atypical features may rarely occur in microglandular hyperplasia and the

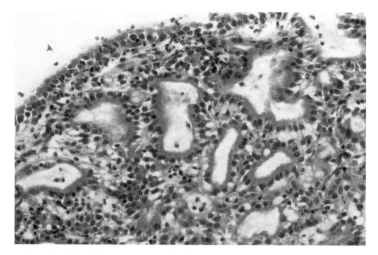

**Fig. 14** Microglandular hyperplasia within the cervix.

absence of a grossly visible mass. The usual differential diagnosis is clear cell carcinoma or endometrial or cervical adenocarcinoma with a microglandular growth pattern. Obviously the presence of severe nuclear atypia or abundant mitotic figures favours a malignant process.

The immunohistochemical panel of MIB1, bcl2, and p16 may be useful in problematic cases. Vimentin positivity favours a microglandular variant of endometrial adenocarcinoma as microglandular hyperplasia is generally negative.[24]

## INTESTINAL METAPLASIA

Intestinal metaplasia involving endocervical crypts has rarely been described.[69] It is characterised by the presence of goblet cells and sometimes Paneth cells and argentaffin cells. In my opinion this is an extremely rare occurrence, if it occurs at all, and most cases represent an intestinal form of CGIN. Two interesting cases have been described in which bland intestinal-type epithelium with goblet cells lined the endometrium and endocervix.[70] Co-existent appendiceal neoplasms were present and differential cytokeratin staining (CK 7 and CK 20) suggested metastasis from the appendix by a transtubal route.

## OXYPHIL METAPLASIA

Oxyphil metaplasia is characterised by replacement of the endocervical cryptal epithelium by cuboidal cells with eosinophilic cytoplasm. Often there is a degree of nuclear atypia and this lesion was originally designated atypical oxyphil metaplasia.[71] Its only significance is that it may be mistaken for CGIN. In my experience, eosinophilic cytoplasm may be seen focally in endocervical crypts, especially in association with inflammation, and a diagnosis of oxyphil metaplasia should be reserved for those rare cases where there is abundant eosinophilic cytoplasm.

45

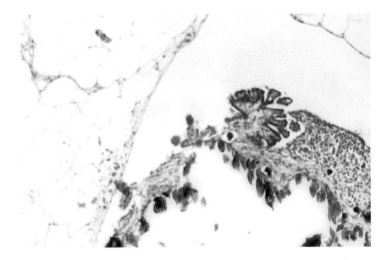

**Fig. 15** Endosalpingiosis involving the omentum. A papillary lesion lined by a single layer of cells is associated with calcified psammoma bodies.

## OTHER MISCELLANEOUS METAPLASIAS WITHIN THE FEMALE GENITAL SYSTEM

Metaplasias elsewhere within the female genital system are relatively rare. In the fallopian tube transitional metaplasia, similar to that seen within the cervix, has been described,[72] and mucinous metaplasia of the fallopian tube has also been reported.[25] There may be an association between mucinous lesions of the fallopian tube, including mucinous metaplasia, and Peutz-Jegher's syndrome. In some cases, multiple mucinous lesions may be present throughout the female genital system, such as mucinous tumours of the ovary or cervix: one patient had a co-existent appendiceal neoplasm.[25] It is difficult to ascertain whether these are synchronous mucinous tumours or metastatic deposits although, in cases with appendiceal pathology, it is likely that CK 7 and CK 20 staining would be of value. Positive CK 20 and negative CK 7 staining in all the lesions would suggest an appendiceal primary with metastatic spread.[73]

The abdominal and pelvic peritoneum, as part of the secondary Müllerian system, may undergo metaplasia into various Müllerian epithelia. The secondary Müllerian system comprises the mesothelium and subjacent mesenchyme of the pelvis and lower abdomen. The Müllerian potential of this tissue is consistent with its close embryonic relation with the Müllerian ducts. Non-neoplastic secondary Müllerian lesions, which are in many cases a form of metaplasia, comprise endometriosis, endosalpingiosis and endocervicosis. When occurring in combination this has been termed Müllerianosis.[74] It is recognised that probably most cases of abdominal and pelvic endometriosis are not truly metaplastic but are the result of retrograde menstruation. Endometriosis will not be described here.

Endosalpingiosis is characterised by the presence of non-neoplastic glands lined by ciliated tubal-type epithelium (Fig. 15).[75] It usually involves the peritoneum and subperitoneal tissues including the surface of the ovaries. Pelvic and retroperitoneal lymph nodes may also be involved. Endosalpingiosis is usually an incidental finding on microscopic examination but rarely may form a

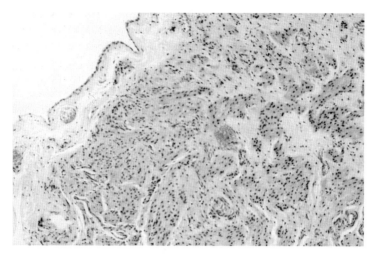

**Fig. 16** Diffuse peritoneal leiomyomatosis composed of bland smooth muscle. A layer of mesothelial cells is present to the left of the photomicrograph.

cystic mass, referred to as florid cystic endosalpingiosis.[76,77] This may involve the serosa of the uterus or cervix. In cases of endosalpingiosis, glands are lined by a single layer of ciliated epithelial cells which exhibit little or no cytological atypia. Psammoma bodies are often present in glandular lumina or the surrounding stroma. Psammoma bodies in the absence of epithelium may indicate atrophic endosalpingiosis. Endosalpingiosis is especially likely to be found in patients with ovarian serous neoplasms which may be benign, borderline or malignant. When associated with such a lesion, endosalpingiosis must not be interpreted as metastatic disease – careful sampling is indicated to exclude co-existent borderline or malignant implants. Occasionally, foci of endosalpingiosis have multilayering with papillary formations and mild cytological atypia. This has been referred to as atypical endosalpingiosis but the distinction from primary peritoneal serous borderline tumours is not clear.[78]

Endocervicosis is characterised histologically by the presence of non-neoplastic mucinous glands resembling endocervical glands. This is much less common than endometriosis or endosalpingiosis. Involved sites have included the peritoneum, pelvic lymph nodes, the urinary bladder, the uterine serosa, the cervix, and the vagina.[74,79–82] Especially when florid and involving the wall of the bladder or cervix, a diagnosis of well-differentiated mucinous adeno-carcinoma, including cervical minimal deviation adenocarcinoma of mucinous type (adenoma malignum), may be considered. The presence of focal atypia or of a reactive stroma may further heighten the resemblance to adenocarcinoma. In the cervix, a useful pointer in distinguishing endocervicosis from adenoma malignum is that in the former the lesion is predominantly situated in the outer aspects of the wall of the cervix. A single case has been described of adeno-carcinoma arising in vaginal endocervicosis.[83]

Another rare metaplastic lesion to arise from the secondary Müllerian system (probably from metaplastic transformation of submesothelial mesenchymal cells) is diffuse peritoneal leiomyomatosis.[84] This condition is characterised by multiple small nodules of bland smooth muscle cells involving the peritoneum and omentum (Fig. 16) and is often associated with pregnancy or exogenous hormones. There may be associated endometriosis, endosalpingiosis or decidualisation. Diffuse peritoneal leiomyomatosis often shows positive immunohistochemical staining with progesterone receptor[85] and persistent cases have been successfully treated with gonadotropin-releasing hormone agonists.[86] Although usually a self-limiting lesion, occasional cases recur (sometimes at the time of subsequent pregnancy) and transformation to leiomyosarcoma has been reported.[87]

---

## Points of best practice

- The Müllerian-derived epithelium which lines most of the female genital system has the capacity to differentiate along a number of pathways resulting in epithelium of ciliated, mucinous, endometrioid, transitional and squamous types. This is also the case with the abdominal and pelvic peritoneum as part of the secondary Müllerian system.

- Endometrial epithelial metaplasias are non-neoplastic lesions.

- With endometrial metaplasias there is a risk of overdiagnosis of malignancy (as these may have a complex architecture) and underdiagnosis of malignancy (as these may co-exist with hyperplasia or carcinoma).

- Endometrial epithelial metaplasias may be associated with exogenous hormone therapy including tamoxifen, an intra-uterine device, chronic endometritis, and pyometra. In many cases there are no known aetiological factors.

- When faced with a cytologically bland endometrial mucinous proliferation with a complex architecture, a diagnosis of well-differentiated mucinous adenocarcinoma should always be considered.

- Cervical tubal metaplasia, tubo-endometrial metaplasia and endometriosis may be mistaken for CGIN. In difficult cases, a panel of immunohistochemical stains (MIB1, bcl2 and p16) may assist in distinguishing these lesions from CGIN. The immunohistochemistry should always be interpreted in the context of the morphological features.

- Cervical microglandular hyperplasia usually has a characteristic histological appearance but atypical features such as stromal hyalinisation, oedema or myxoid change, signet-ring or spindle-shaped cells, solid or trabecular areas and nuclear pleomorphism may occasionally result in diagnostic difficulties.

---

### References

1. *Stedman's Medical Dictionary*, 24 edn. Baltimore, MD; Williams and Wilkins, 1982; 864.
2. Lauchlan SC. Metaplasias and neoplasias of Müllerian epithelium. *Histopathology* 1984; **8**: 543–557.

3. Kennedy MM, Baigrie CF, Manek S. Tamoxifen and the endometrium: review of 102 cases and comparison with HRT-related and non-HRT-related endometrial pathology. *Int J Gynecol Pathol* 1999; **18**: 130–137.

4. Ismail SM. Pathology of endometrium treated with tamoxifen. *J Clin Pathol* 1994; **47**: 827–833.

5. McCluggage WG, Desai V, Manek S. Tamoxifen-associated postmenopausal adenomyosis exhibits stromal fibrosis, glandular dilatation and epithelial metaplasia. *Histopathology* 2000; **37**: 340–346.

6. Young RH, Scully RE. Uterine carcinomas simulating microglandular hyperplasia. A report of six cases. *Am J Surg Pathol* 1992; **16**: 1092–1097.

7. Zaloudek C, Hayashi GM, Ryan IP, Bethan Powell C, Miller TM. Microglandular adenocarcinoma of the endometrium. A form of mucinous adenocarcinoma that may be confused with microglandular hyperplasia of the cervix. *Int J Gynecol Pathol* 1999; **16**: 52–59.

8. McCluggage WG, Perenyei M. Microglandular adenocarcinoma of the endometrium. *Histopathology* 2000; **37**: 285–287.

9. Hendrickson MR, Kempson RL. Endometrial epithelial metaplasias: proliferations frequently misdiagnosed as adenocarcinoma. Report of 89 cases and proposed classification. *Am J Surg Pathol* 1980; **4**: 525–542.

10. Kaku T, Tsukamoto N, Tsuruchi N *et al*. Endometrial metaplasia associated with endometrial carcinoma. *Obstet Gynecol* 1992; **80**: 812–816.

11. Anderson WA, Taylor Jr PT, Fechner RE, Pinkerton JA. Endometrial metaplasia associated with endometrial adenocarcinoma. *Am J Obstet Gynecol* 1987; **157**: 597–604.

12. Zaino RJ, Kurman RJ. Squamous differentiation in carcinoma of the endometrium: critical appraisal of adenocanthoma and adenosquamous carcinoma. *Semin Diagn Pathol* 1988; **5**: 154–171.

13. Clement PB, Young RH. Endometrioid carcinoma of the uterine corpus: a review of its pathology with emphasis on recent advances and problematic aspects. *Adv Anat Pathol* 2002; **9**: 145–184.

14. Longacre TA, Chung MH, Rouse RV, Hendrickson MR. Atypical polypoid adenomyofibromas (atypical polypoid adenomyomas) of the uterus. A clinicopathologic study of 55 cases. *Am J Surg Pathol* 1996; **20**: 1–20.

15. Mazur MT. Atypical polypoid adenomyomas of the endometrium. *Am J Surg Pathol* 1981; **5**: 473–482.

16. Young RH, Treger T, Scully RE. Atypical polypoid adenomyoma of the uterus. A report of 27 cases. *Am J Clin Pathol* 1986; **86**: 139–145.

17. Miranda MC, Mazur MT. Endometrial squamous metaplasia. An unusual response to progestin therapy of hyperplasia. *Arch Pathol Lab Med* 1995; **119**: 458–460.

18. Mount ML. Mucinous metaplasias of the endometrium: biologically meaningful subsets for the practising surgical pathologist. *Adv Anat Pathol* 2000; **7**: 197–200.

19. Wells M, Tiltman A. Intestinal metaplasia of the endometrium. *Histopathology* 1989; **15**: 431–433.

20. McCluggage WG, Roberts N, Bharucha H. Enteric differentiation in endometrial adenocarcinomas: a mucin histochemical study. *Int J Gynecol Pathol* 1995; **14**: 250–254.

21. Savargaonkar PR, Hale RT, Pope R, Fox H, Buckley H. Enteric differentiation in cervical adenocarcinomas and its prognostic significance. *Histopathology* 1993; **23**: 275–277.

22. Nucci MR, Prasad CJ, Crum CP, Mutter GL. Mucinous endometrial epithelial proliferations: a morphologic spectrum of changes with diverse clinical significance. *Mod Pathol* 1999; **12**: 1137–1142.

23. Jacques SM, Qureshi F, Lawrence WD. Surface epithelial changes in endometrial adenocarcinoma: diagnostic pitfalls in curettage specimens. *Int J Gynecol Pathol* 1995; **14**: 191–197.

24. Qiu W, Mittal K. Comparison of morphologic and immunostaining patterns of cervical microglandular hyperplasia with low nuclear grade mucinous adenocarcinoma of the endometrium. *Mod Pathol* 2002; **15**: 207A.

25. Seidman JD. Mucinous lesions of the fallopian tube. A report of seven cases. *Am J Surg Pathol* 1994; **18**: 1205–1212.

26. Hendrickson MR, Kempson RL. Ciliated carcinoma – a variant of endometrial adenocarcinoma: a report of 10 cases. *Int J Gynecol Pathol* 1983; **2**: 1–12.

27. Silver SA, Cheung ANY, Tavassoli FA. Oncocytic metaplasia and carcinoma of the endometrium: an immunohistochemical and ultrastructural study. *Int J Gynecol Pathol* 1989; **18**: 12–19.

28. Pitman MB, Young RH, Clement PB, Dickersin GR, Scully RE. Endometrioid carcinoma of the ovary and endometrium, oxyphilic cell type: a report of nine cases. *Int J Gynecol Pathol* 1994; **13**: 290–301.

29. Zaman SS, Mazur MT. Endometrial papillary syncytial change: a non-specific alteration associated with active breakdown. *Am J Clin Pathol* 1993; **99**: 741–745.

30. Lehman MB, Hart WR. Simple and complex hyperplastic papillary proliferations of the endometrium: a clinicopathologic study of nine cases of apparently localised papillary lesions with fibrovascular stromal cores and epithelial metaplasia. *Am J Surg Pathol* 2001; **25**: 1347–1354.

31. Arias-Stella J. Atypical endometrial changes associated with the presence of chorionic tissue. *Arch Pathol Lab Med* 1954; **58**: 112–128.

32. Huettner PC, Gersell DJ. Arias-Stella reaction in non pregnant women: a clinicopathologic study of nine cases. *Int J Gynecol Pathol* 1994; **13**: 241–247.

33. Arias-Stella Jr J, Arias-Velasquez A, Arias-Stella J. Normal and abnormal mitoses in the atypical endometrial change associated with chorionic tissue effect. *Am J Surg Pathol* 1994; **18**: 694–701.

34. Arias-Stella J. The Arias-Stella reaction: facts and fancies four decades after. *Adv Anat Pathol* 2002; **9**: 12–23.

35. Bird CC, Willis RA. The production of smooth muscle by the endometrial stroma of the adult human uterus. *J Pathol Bacteriol* 1965; **90**: 75–81.

36. McCluggage WG, Sumathi VP, Maxwell P. CD10 is a sensitive and diagnostically useful immunohistochemical marker of normal endometrial stroma and of endometrial stromal neoplasms. *Histopathology* 2001; **39**: 273–278.

37. Franquemont DW, Frierson Jr HF, Mills SE. An immunohistochemical study of normal endometrial stroma and endometrial stromal neoplasms: evidence for smooth muscle differentiation. *Am J Surg Pathol* 1991; **15**: 861–870.

38. Oliva E, Clement PB, Young RH, Scully RE. Mixed endometrial stromal and smooth muscle tumors of the uterus: a clinicopathologic study of 15 cases. *Am J Surg Pathol* 1998; **22**: 997–1005.

39. Ganem KJ, Parsons L, Friedell GH. Endometrial ossification. *Am J Obstet Gynecol* 1962; **83**: 1592–1594.

40. Bahceci M, Demirel LC. Osseous metaplasia of the endometrium: a rare cause of infertility and it hysteroscopic management. *Hum Reprod* 1996; **11**: 2537–2539.

41. Roth E, Taylor HB, Heterotopic cartilage in uterus. *Obstet Gynecol* 1966; **27**: 838–844.

42. Nogales FF, Gomez-Morales M, Raymundo C, Aguilar D. Benign heterologous tissue components associated with endometrial carcinoma. *Int J Gynecol Pathol* 1982; **1**: 286–291.

43. Gronroos M, Meurman L, Kahra K. Proliferating glia and other heterotopic tissues in the uterus: fetal homografts? *Obstet Gynecol* 1983; **61**: 261–266.

44. Rocca AN, Guajardo M, Estrada WJ. Glial polyp of the cervix and endometrium. *Am J Clin Pathol* 1980; **73**: 718–720.

45. Nogales FF, Pavcovich M, Medina MT, Palomino M. Fatty change in the endometrium. *Histopathology* 1992; **20**: 599–600.

46. McCluggage WG, Hamal P, Traub AI, Walsh MY. Uterine adenolipoleiomyoma: a rare hamartomatous lesion. *Int J Gynecol Pathol* 2000; **19**: 183–185.

47. Cregh TM, Bain BJ, Evans DJ *et al*. Endometrial extramedullary haemopoiesis. *J Pathol* 1995; **176**: 99–104.

48. Sirgi KE, Swanson PE, Gersell DJ. Extramedullary haematopoiesis in the endometrium: report of four cases and review of the literature. *Am J Clin Pathol* 1994; **101**: 643–646.

49. Valeri RM, Ibrahim N, Sheaff MT. Extramedullary haematopoiesis in the endometrium. *Int J Gynecol Pathol* 2002; **21**: 178–181.

50. Crum CP, Egawa K, Fu YS *et al*. Atypical immature metaplasia (AIM). A subset of human papilloma virus infection of the cervix. *Cancer* 1983; **51**: 2214–2219.

51. Park JJ, Genest DR, Sun D, Crum CP. Atypical immature metaplastic-like proliferations of the cervix: diagnostic reproducibility and viral (HPV) correlates. *Hum Pathol* 1999; **30**: 1161–1165.

52. Park JJ, Sun D, Quade BJ *et al*. Stratified mucin-producing intraepithelial lesions of the cervix. Adenosquamous or columnar cell neoplasia? *Am J Surg Pathol* 2000; **24**: 1414–1419.

53. Egan AJM, Russell P. Transitional (urothelial) cell metaplasia of the uterine cervix: morphological assessment of 31 cases. *Int J Gynecol Pathol* 1997; **16**: 89–98.

54. Weir MM, Beu DA, Young RH. Transitional cell metaplasia of the uterine cervix and vagina: an underrecognised lesion that may be confused with high-grade dysplasia. *Am J Surg Pathol* 1997; **21**: 510–517.

55. Miller N, Bebard YC, Cooter NB, Shaul DL. Histological changes in the genital tract in transsexual women following androgen therapy. *Histopathology* 1986; **10**: 661–669.

56. Weir MM, Bell DA. Transitional cell metaplasia of the cervix: a newly described entity in cervicovaginal smears. *Diagn Cytopathol* 1998; **18**: 222–226.

57. Harnden P, Kennedy W, Andrew AC, Southgate J. Immunophenotype of transitional metaplasia of the uterine cervix. *Int J Gynecol Pathol* 1999; **18**: 125–129.

58. Ismail SM. Cone biopsy causes cervical endometriosis and tuboendometrioid metaplasia. *Histopathology* 1991; **18**: 107–114.

59. Al-Nafussi A, Rahilly M. The prevalence of tuboendometrial metaplasia and adenomatoid proliferation. *Histopathology* 1993; **22**: 177–179.

60. Baker PM, Clement PB, Bell DA, Young RH. Superficial endometriosis of the uterine cervix: a report of 20 cases of a process that may be confused with endocervical glandular dysplasia or adenocarcinoma *in situ*. Int J Gynecol Pathol 1999; **18**: 198–205.

61. Oliva E, Clement PB, Young RH. Tubal and tubo-endometrioid metaplasia of the uterine cervix. Unemphasised features that may cause problems in differential diagnosis. A report of 25 cases. *Am J Clin Pathol* 1995; **103**: 618–623.

62. Schlesinger C, Silverberg SG. Endocervical adenocarcinoma *in situ* of tubal type and its relation to atypical tubal metaplasia. *Int J Gynecol Pathol* 1999; **18**: 1–4.

63. Cameron RI, Maxwell P, Jenkins D, McCluggage WG. Immunohistochemical staining with MIB1, bcl-2 and p16 assists in the distinction of cervical glandular intraepithelial neoplasia from tubo-endometrial metaplasia, endometriosis and microglandular hyperplasia. *Histopathology* 2002; **41**: 313–321.

64. McCluggage WG, Maxwell P, McBride HA, Hamilton PW, Bharucha H. Monoclonal antibodies Ki-67 and MIB1 in the distinction of tuboendometrial metaplasia from endocervical adenocarcinoma and adenocarcinoma *in situ* in formalin-fixed material. *Int J Gynecol Pathol* 1995; **14**: 209–216.

65. McCluggage WG, Maxwell P, Bharucha H. Immunohistochemical detection of p53 and bcl-2 in neoplastic and non-neoplastic endocervical glandular lesions. *Int J Gynecol Pathol* 1997; **16**: 22–27.

66. McCluggage WG, Maxwell P. Bcl-2 and p21 immunostaining of cervical tubo-endometrial metaplasia. *Histopathology* 2002; **40**: 107–108.

67. Greeley C, Schroeder S, Silverberg SG. Microglandular hyperplasia of the cervix: a true 'pill' lesion? *Int J Gynecol Pathol* 1995; **14**: 50–54.

68. Young RH, Scully RE. Atypical forms of microglandular hyperplasia of the cervix simulating carcinoma: a report of five cases and review of the literature. *Am J Surg Pathol* 1989; **13**: 50–56.

69. Trowell JE. Intestinal metaplasia with argentaffin cells in the uterine cervix. *Histopathology* 1985; **9**: 551–559.

70. Moore WF, Bentley RC, Kim KR, Olatidoye B, Gray SR, Robboy SJ. Goblet-cell mucinous epithelium lining the endometrium and endocervix: evidence of metastasis from an appendiceal primary tumor through the use of cytokeratin-7 and –20 immunostains. *Int J Gynecol Pathol* 1998; **17**: 363–367.

71. Jones MA, Young RH. Atypical oxyphilic metaplasia of the endocervical epithelium: a report of six cases. *Int J Gynecol Pathol* 1997; **16**: 99–102.

72. Egan AJM, Russell P. Transitional (urothelial) metaplasia of the fallopian tube mucosa: morphological assessment of three cases. *Int J Gynecol Pathol* 1996; **15**: 72–76.

73. McCluggage WG. Recent advances in immunohistochemistry in gynaecological pathology. *Histopathology* 2002; **40**: 309–326.

74. Young RH, Clement PB. Müllerianosis of the urinary bladder. *Mod Pathol* 1996; **9**: 731–737.

75. Zinsser KR. Endosalpingiosis in the omentum. A study of autopsy and surgical material. *Am J Surg Pathol* 1982; **6**: 109–117.

76. Clement PB, Young RH. Florid cystic endosalpingiosis with tumor-like manifestations. A report of four cases including the first reported cases of transmural endosalpingiosis of the uterus. *Am J Surg Pathol* 1999; **23**: 166–175.

77. McCluggage WG, Weir PE. Paraovarian cystic endosalpingiosis in association with tamoxifen therapy. *J Clin Pathol* 2000; **53**: 161–162.

78. Bell DA, Scully RE. Serous borderline tumors of the peritoneum. *Am J Surg Pathol* 1990; **14**: 230–239.

79. Nazeer T, Ro JY, Tornos C *et al.* Endocervical type glands in urinary bladder: a clinicopathologic study of six cases. *Hum Pathol* 1996; **27**: 816–820.

80. Clement PB, Young RH. Endocervicosis of the urinary bladder: a report of six cases of a benign Müllerian lesion that may mimic adenocarcinoma. *Am J Surg Pathol* 1992; **16**: 533–542.

81. Young RH, Clement PB. Endocervicosis involving the uterine cervix: a report of four cases of a benign process that may be confused with deeply invasive endocervical adenocarcinoma. *Int J Gynecol Pathol* 2000; **19**: 322–328.

82. Martiaka M, Allaire C, Clement PB. Endocervicosis presenting as a painful vaginal mass: a case report. *Int J Gynecol Pathol* 1999; **18**: 274–276.

83. McCluggage WG, Price JH, Dobbs SP. Primary adenocarcinoma of the vagina arising in endocervicosis. *Int J Gynecol Pathol* 2001; **20**: 399–402.

84. Tavassoli FA, Norris HJ. Peritoneal leiomyomatosis (leiomyomatosis peritonealis disseminata): a clinicopathologic study of 20 cases with ultrastructural observations. *Int J Gynecol Pathol* 1982; **1**: 59–74.

85. Butnor KJ, Burchette JL, Robboy SJ. Progesterone receptor activity in leiomyomatosis peritonealis disseminata. *Int J Gynecol Pathol* 1999; **18**: 259–264.

86. Clavero PA, Nogales FF, Ruiz-Avila I *et al.* Regression of peritoneal leiomyomatosis after treatment with gonadotropin releasing hormone analogue. *Int J Gynecol Cancer* 1992; **2**: 52–54.

87. Abulafia O, Angel C, Sherer DM *et al.* Computed tomography of leiomyomatosis peritonealis disseminata with malignant transformation. *Am J Obstet Gynecol* 1995; **189**: 52–54.

*David N. Slater*

4

# Classification and diagnosis of cutaneous lymphoproliferative diseases

This chapter describes the main advances in cutaneous lymphoproliferative diseases that have occurred since the topic last received consideration in *Recent Advances in Histopathology*.[1] In particular, it provides general guidance on the diagnosis of cutaneous lymphoma and highlights diagnostic pitfalls. In addition, it describes the new World Health Organization (WHO) classification of haematopoietic and lymphoid tissues, as applied to the skin.[2]

## GENERAL GUIDANCE ON THE DIAGNOSIS OF CUTANEOUS LYMPHOMA

### THE MULTIDISCIPLINARY TEAM

The key to the correct diagnosis of cutaneous lymphoma lies in interspecialty communication. As primary cutaneous lymphoma is so rare, all cases should be reviewed by designated specialists and discussed by a multidisciplinary team. Cutaneous lymphoma has been defined by the Department of Health as requiring specialised histopathology and dermatology services, with the associated implication for central referral.

### THE DIAGNOSTIC GOLD STANDARD

The underlying principle in the diagnosis of cutaneous lymphoma is that no solitary diagnostic gold standard exists and that an accurate diagnosis can be achieved only by the amalgamation of several diagnostic variables. As a minimum, these must include clinical features, the histopathological appearance and the immunophenotype of the lymphoma. Molecular investigations make an increasing contribution and should be available to those diagnosing cutaneous

**Dr David Neil Slater** MBChB BMSci FRCPath
Consultant Dermatopathologist, Royal Hallamshire Hospital, Glossop Road, Sheffield S10 4LA, UK
E-mail: david.slater@sth.nhs.uk

lymphoproliferative diseases. In addition, the functional biology of the neoplastic cells and aetiological factors, such as human T-cell leukaemia virus and Epstein-Barr virus, can be relevant to the diagnosis. Each of these will be discussed separately.

## CLINICOPATHOLOGICAL CORRELATION

The chance of diagnostic disaster is high when the histopathologist who reports cutaneous lymphoma does so in the absence of full clinical information. Request forms often have insufficient detail and although patients' notes can be helpful, each case should be discussed with a clinician. For histopathologists with experience in clinical dermatology, the best approach is clinicopathological correlation based on personal examination of the patient.

The distinction between primary and secondary cutaneous lymphoma has major therapeutic and prognostic implications. Excluding mycosis fungoides and Sézary syndrome, the European Organization for the Research and Treatment of Cancer (EORTC) defined primary cutaneous lymphoma as one presenting in the skin with no evidence of extracutaneous disease within the first 6 months.[3] In most centres, however, this definition has been superseded by negative staging at the time of presentation, including imaging and bone marrow trephine biopsy.

A potentially confusing clinical feature is the phenomenon of spontaneous lesional regression in some cutaneous lymphomas, illustrating that regression is not purely the prerogative of reactive conditions.

## HISTOPATHOLOGICAL LIMITATIONS

Histopathologists must resist requests to diagnose cutaneous lymphoma on punch biopsies and instead encourage clinicians to ensure that biopsies are of a reasonable size and extend into subcutaneous adipose tissue. Many cutaneous lymphomas evolve over a long time and some histopathological features may initially not be present. This is one reason why cutaneous lymphoma can be difficult to diagnose and may require multiple sequential biopsies before the diagnosis is established. Review of previous biopsies is also essential in this situation.

A vital skill of the histopathologist is the art of disease recognition by pattern analysis. In cutaneous lymphoma, however, although pattern analysis is useful, no pattern is specific to any one disease or cell lineage. The best achievable result is usually a short differential diagnosis of diseases or cell types that can be associated with the pattern present. For example, epidermotropism is characteristic of many T-cell infiltrates, but does not permit a distinction between a reactive and a neoplastic process. In addition, epidermotropism may be observed occasionally in B-cell infiltrates and with other cell types, such as in Langerhans' cell histiocytosis. Conversely, a non-epidermotropic pattern is often seen in neoplastic B-cell infiltrates but can also occur with neoplastic T-cell infiltrates. The intra-epidermal collection of lymphocytes and antigen-presenting cells (designated a Pautrier abscess or micro-abscess) is often considered pathogonomic of mycosis fungoides. It can, however, be seen in other types of cutaneous T-cell lymphoma and can be mimicked by collections of epithelial cells as in neuro-endocrine carcinoma. Angiocentricity, angiodestruction and coagulative necrosis are common features of natural killer (NK) cell lymphomas but are also characteristic of lymphomatoid granulomatosis. Granulomas can be seen in granulomatous slack disease and lymphomatoid granulomatosis but are a stromal reaction in many types of cutaneous lymphoma.

## IMMUNOPHENOTYPIC ANALYSIS

Most relevant antibodies now work on paraffin sections where frozen sections were previously required. Caution should be exercised in comparing scientific publications that have used different methodologies. For example, this is the probable explanation for the reports of variable CD10 expression in follicular cutaneous B-cell lymphoma.

The antibodies used should include those for T cells (CD2, CD3 and CD45RO), their subtypes (helper/inducer CD4 and cytotoxic/suppressor CD8), B cells (CD20 and CD79a), their subtypes (CD5, CD10 and bcl-6), NK cells (CD56 and CD57), histiocytes (CD68), and dendritic cells (S100, CD1a, CD21, CD23 and factor 13a). Blast cells should be stained for CD30 and, if positive, for ALK-1 protein. Other antibodies include those for bcl-2, nuclear proliferation (Ki67), cyclin D1 and cytotoxic function (T-cell intracellular antigen – TIA-1, granzyme B and perforin). Immunohistochemistry to demonstrate light-chain restriction can be helpful, but is often capricious. Family-specific antibodies against the V-beta T-cell receptor (TCR) gene can provide a useful clonotypic marker in cutaneous T-cell lymphoma. These do not currently cover all families and may not identify all gene segments for a specific family.

In most cases, immunohistochemistry can identify the cell lineage of the neoplastic cells. Difficulties can arise because neoplasms contain not only neoplastic but also reactive lymphoid cells. In some cases, the neoplastic cells may be present in only small numbers and can be mistaken for the reactive cell population. Examples include T-cell/histiocyte-rich follicular cutaneous B-cell lymphoma and lymphomatoid granulomatosis.

Different types of cutaneous T-cell lymphoma tend to be associated with a more frequent T-cell subtype though this is never absolute. Mycosis fungoides, for example, though usually of CD4 helper/inducer type, can occasionally be of CD8 cytotoxic/suppressor type. Depending on the type of lymphoma, a subtype (such as CD8) can be associated with either a good or poor prognosis. Phenotypic aberrance and loss of antigens can be useful in the diagnosis of cutaneous T-cell lymphoma, but it is not a consistent abnormality.

## MOLECULAR INVESTIGATIONS

Genotypic analysis to assess clonality has made a significant contribution to cutaneous lymphoma during the last decade. In particular, it has allowed the nosological status of various entities to be defined more accurately. For example, many putative B-cell pseudolymphomas are now recognised to be follicular cutaneous B-cell lymphomas; regressing atypical histiocytosis, granulomatous slack skin disease and pagetoid reticulosis are examples of cutaneous T-cell lymphoma. The contribution of genotypic analysis to the diagnosis, staging, prognostic evaluation and management of patients with cutaneous lymphoproliferative diseases supports the view that access to this facility should now be regarded as a standard quality of care.

Southern blot analysis has been largely superseded by techniques based on the polymerase chain reaction (PCR). This is more sensitive and can often be used on material embedded in paraffin wax. The most useful application of PCR is the assessment of clonality in T and B cells by investigating potential re-arrangement of the TCR or B-cell immunoglobulin heavy-chain genes.

The sensitivity of PCR permits the demonstration of monoclonality in a significant proportion of early cases of cutaneous T-cell lymphoma and follicular cutaneous B-cell lymphoma and can reduce the number of equivocal histopathology reports. It has also been proposed that the presence of a peripheral blood T-cell monoclone should be a pre-requisite for the diagnosis of Sézary syndrome.[4] The presence of a T-cell monoclone in a lymph node or peripheral blood of a patient with cutaneous T-cell lymphoma contributes important staging and prognostic information.[5] Furthermore, it can contribute to our knowledge of tumour burden and therapeutic response.[6]

It is essential, however, that some limitations of genotypic analysis are appreciated. The biological implication of clonality is not absolute: polyclonality and monoclonality do not always correlate with reactive and neoplastic diseases, respectively and both can be associated with benign or malignant biological behaviour. Monoclonal T cells have been occasionally detected in the peripheral blood of healthy elderly patients and in the cutaneous infiltrates of various diseases including pityriasis lichenoides, lichen sclerosus, lichen planus, and pigmented purpuric dermatosis. The sensitivity of PCR has led to the emergence of new molecular disease diagnoses such as clonal dermatitis.

The re-arrangement of the alpha-beta or gamma-delta TCR genes are not specific to one type of cutaneous T-cell lymphoma and may have different prognostic and therapeutic implications. For example, lymphomas derived from gamma-delta T-cells are usually CD4 and CD8 negative and tend to have a worse prognosis. The PCR results can have false negatives and false positives. Some of these may be due to technical problems of quality control; others may be associated with the disease itself, such as somatic hypermutation and false negative results in follicular cutaneous B-cell lymphoma.[7] In summary, the findings of genotypic analysis must always be interpreted in the clinical and histopathological context.

By comparison, cytogenetic analysis has proved to be less diagnostically useful. For example, t(14;18) translocation is absent in many cases of primary follicular cutaneous B-cell lymphoma and the frequency of trisomy 3, t(11;18) and t(1;14) in primary marginal zone follicular cutaneous B-cell lymphoma remains uncertain. Studies in cutaneous T-cell lymphoma have shown variable findings but with a common theme of abnormalities on chromosomes 9 and 10.[8]

As in other malignancies, candidate tumour suppressor genes have been identified in cutaneous lymphoma. Mutations of p53 have been identified as a marker of disease progression in the tumour stage of mycosis fungoides.[9]

These can be of a type associated with ultraviolet (UV) light exposure,[9] but the effect of previous phototherapy is unclear. There is increasing evidence of inactivation of the p15 and p16 genes in both cutaneous T-cell lymphoma and follicular cutaneous B-cell lymphoma.[10-12] These are located on chromosome region 9p21 and are inactivated by either allelic loss or hypermethylation of the promotor regions. Their functional loss can be demonstrated by immunohistochemistry and this may be of diagnostic use.

DNA microarrays and gene expression profiling can identify distinct molecular subtypes of nodal lymphoma that appear clinically important.[13] It seems likely that this methodology will eventually have great importance in the classification of cutaneous lymphoma.

## BIOLOGICAL BEHAVIOUR

In some instances, cutaneous lymphoma can be subclassified by the demonstration of granule-associated cytotoxic activity using antibodies to granzyme B, perforin or TIA-1. In addition, cutaneous T-cell lymphoma can be subdivided according to the pattern of cytokine production: Sézary syndrome, for example, is usually caused by Th2 cells.

## THE CLASSIFICATION OF CUTANEOUS LYMPHOMA

The classification of nodal and extranodal lymphoma has undergone substantial change in the last decade and the Revised European-American Lymphoma (REAL) classification was the first to be based on distinctive clinicopathological entities.[14] For cutaneous lymphoma, however, greatest emphasis has been given to the EORTC classification.[3] Similar to REAL, it bases diagnoses on a combination of clinical, histological, immunohistochemical and genetic criteria. It remains the only classification dedicated purely to primary cutaneous lymphoma and continues to have substantial support. This is because of its capacity to define specific cutaneous diseases with distinct clinical and histological features, including a predictable clinical course, response to therapy and prognosis. The EORTC classification has been subject to criticism, especially in respect of follicular cutaneous B-cell lymphoma. This relates especially to the EORTC category of primary cutaneous follicular centre cell lymphoma, which is not homogeneous and incorporates REAL examples of follicular lymphoma, marginal zone lymphoma and diffuse large B-cell lymphoma.[15,16]

## THE WHO CLASSIFICATION OF TUMOURS OF HAEMATOPOIETIC AND LYMPHOID TISSUES

The WHO classification of tumours of haematopoietic and lymphoid tissues evolved from meetings at Orlando and Virginia and cumulated in a recent publication in the WHO Blue Book series.[2,17,18] The classification represents the first world-wide consensus classification of lymphoid and haematopoietic neoplasms. The WHO classification has adopted the same concept as REAL and defines disease entities based on a combination of morphology, immunophenotypic, genetic and clinical features. The underlying principle is again that no one variable must be regarded as a diagnostic gold standard. Some diseases are defined by morphology with immunophenotypic backup, whereas in others clinical features or a genetic abnormality are more important.

## THE WHO CLASSIFICATION AND CUTANEOUS LYMPHOMA

With reference to the skin, WHO divides lymphoid tissues into those of B-, T- and NK-cell types. There are also entries for myeloproliferative and myelodysplastic disorders, histiocyte and dendritic cell neoplasms, Hodgkin lymphoma and mastocytosis. A crucial aspect of the classification is the recommendation from the WHO advisory committees that clinical grouping according to prognosis and treatment of organ-related lymphomas, such as the skin, is not necessary. Instead, clinicians and pathologists are directed to become acquainted with each disease entity, its morphology and clinical behaviour. Pathologists are advised to provide free-text explanatory comments in their reports. Although this approach has the benefit of a common language and better interspecialty communication, it could be regarded as suboptimal for the skin. Many primary cutaneous lymphomas are distinctive, often have an indolent course and require special management and therapeutic consideration. From this perspective, it is understandable that the EORTC would wish to defend its clinically relevant organ-based classification.

Compared with REAL, the number of primary cutaneous diseases in the WHO classification has significantly increased. Mycosis fungoides, Sézary syndrome, T-cell primary cutaneous anaplastic large cell lymphoma and subcutaneous panniculitis-like T-cell lymphoma appear as specific entities. Lymphomatoid papulosis, post-transplant lymphoproliferative diseases and lymphomatoid granulomatosis appear under the new categories of T- and B-cell proliferations of uncertain malignant potential. It is noteworthy that follicular cutaneous B-cell lymphoma has not received recognition in the coded summary classification, although cutaneous follicular centre lymphoma is acknowledged within the text to be a specific disease variant. Instead, pathologists are instructed to describe the distinctive features of follicular centre cutaneous B-cell lymphoma. Primary cutaneous CD30 positive T-cell lymphoproliferative disorders have a stand-alone chapter but are then split and separated in the coded summary classification. This displays no CD30-positive qualification for primary cutaneous anaplastic large cell lymphoma; this is only defined in the main text.

Despite the attractions of a stand-alone skin lymphoma classification, the international way forward will be to use the WHO classification. Indeed, The Royal College of Pathologists has adopted the WHO classification for its minimum dataset for the histopathological reporting of lymphoma. Skin has been allocated a specimen type entry and there is a requirement to record the biopsy site as this may influence clinical management and prognosis.[19]

Despite this, it is easy to envisage variable practice in the application of the WHO classification to the skin. The Royal College of Pathologists' minimum dataset contains no specific guidance to the skin, so I propose ways in which the WHO classification could be applied to the skin in a consistent manner.

As recommended by the WHO, The Royal College of Pathologists' minimum dataset contains a free-text comment section to permit the histopathologist to provide guidance on likely biological behaviour. In

**Table 1** Principal primary and secondary cutaneous lymphoproliferative diseases in the WHO summary classification

**B-cell neoplasms**
    Precursor B-lymphoblastic leukaemia/lymphoma
    Chronic lymphocytic leukaemia/small lymphocytic lymphoma
    Lymphoplasmacytic lymphoma/Waldenstrom's macroglobulinaemia
    Hairy cell leukaemia
    Plasma cell myeloma
    Extraosseous plasmacytoma
    Extranodal marginal zone B-cell lymphoma of mucosa-associated
        lymphoid tissue (MALT-lymphoma)
    Follicular lymphoma
        Variants:      Cutaneous follicular centre lymphoma
                     Diffuse follicle centre lymphoma
    Mantle cell lymphoma
    Diffuse large B-cell lymphoma
    Intravascular large B-cell lymphoma
    *Cutaneous B-cell lymphoma, unspecified*

**B-cell proliferations of uncertain malignant potential**
    Lymphomatoid granulomatosis
    Post-transplant lymphoproliferative disorder, polymorphic

**T-cell and NK-cell neoplasms**
    Precursor T-lymphoblastic leukaemia/lymphoma
    Blastic NK-cell lymphoma
    Adult T-cell leukaemia/lymphoma
    Extranodal NK/T-cell lymphoma, nasal type
    Subcutaneous panniculitis-like T-cell lymphoma
    Mycosis fungoides
        Variants:      Pagetoid reticulosis (Woringer-Kolopp disease)
                     Mycosis fungoides – associated follicular mucinosis
                     Granulomatous slack skin disease
    Sézary syndrome
    Primary cutaneous anaplastic large cell lymphoma
        CD30 positive
    Peripheral T-cell lymphoma
        *Primary cutaneous CD30-positive non-anaplastic large cell lymphoma*
        *Primary cutaneous CD30-negative anaplastic and non-anaplastic large*
            *cell lymphoma*
        *Primary cutaneous CD30-negative pleomorphic small/medium cell lymphoma*
        *Primary cutaneous CD56-positive NK-like T-cell lymphomas*
        *Primary cutaneous T-cell lymphoma, unspecified*
    Angioimmunoblastic T-cell lymphoma
    Anaplastic large cell lymphoma
        Secondary cutaneous involvement by systemic anaplastic large
            cell lymphoma (ALCL)

**T-cell proliferation of uncertain malignant potential**
    Lymphomatoid papulosis

**Hodgkin lymphoma**

*Italics,* areas of clarification suggested by the author to facilitate more consistent application of the classification for data collection and research.

particular, this relates to instances in which there is a danger of clinically indolent disease receiving over-treatment for a high-grade histological appearance. To a degree this goes some way to satisfying critics who claim that the WHO classification is less clinically relevant than that of the EORTC. The Royal College of Pathologists' minimum dataset permits other information to be included in the report such as immunophenotypic and genotypic analysis.

Elaboration appears necessary in two areas of the WHO classification. Variants of cutaneous lymphoma appear to exist but are not recognised by the WHO as they fall below their stringent criteria to warrant formal classification. To facilitate research, it seems desirable that data relating to those entities are collected in a consistent manner. Some cutaneous B-cell lymphomas are of uncertain pathogenetic origin and a category of 'CBCL-unspecified' appears desirable. In particular, there can be mixed features of marginal zone and follicular cutaneous B-cell lymphoma to an extent that one might consider a common origin.

Table 1 lists the principal headings in the WHO coded summary classification that are most relevant to primary and secondary cutaneous lymphoma. It incorporates clarifications to facilitate the consistent application of the classification. Some classifications are from the main text of the WHO classification; those in italics are my own suggestions.

I have not attempted to discuss all of the diseases in Table 1 as this has been achieved by the WHO and EORTC publications. A detailed comparison of the two classifications is available.[20] Instead, I will discuss those primary cutaneous diseases warranting special comment, clarification or elaboration.

## B-CELL LYMPHOPROLIFERATIVE DISEASES

### MARGINAL ZONE LYMPHOMA

After considerable controversy, it is now accepted that marginal zone lymphoma can occur in the skin as primary follicular cutaneous B-cell lymphoma.[21,22] Defining molecular criteria have yet to be fully established, but the morphology and immunophenotype usually permit distinction from follicular lymphoma. This could be viewed as academic as these two types of primary cutaneous B-cell lymphoma are clinically similar. Both commonly present on the head, neck and trunk and have the same good prognosis.

Except for a relative paucity of lympho-epithelial lesions, the features of marginal zone lymphoma in the skin are identical to those in other extranodal sites. The infiltrate has a prominence of small cells and appears polymorphous with a combination of plasma cells, centrocyte-like and monocytoid cells. The follicular mantles are often enlarged and germinal centres can show reactive changes with tingible-body macrophages (Fig. 1). The immunophenotype is characteristically CD5- and CD10-negative and the CD21 follicular dendritic network is usually expanded. Neoplastic lymphocytes can be CD23-positive.

Confusion with follicular lymphoma can arise in several ways. The colonisation of germinal centres by neoplastic cells in marginal zone lymphoma can morphologically mimic follicular lymphoma: reactive germinal centres will contain CD10- and bcl-6-positive cells and the neoplastic cells in cutaneous marginal zone lymphoma are often bcl-2-positive.

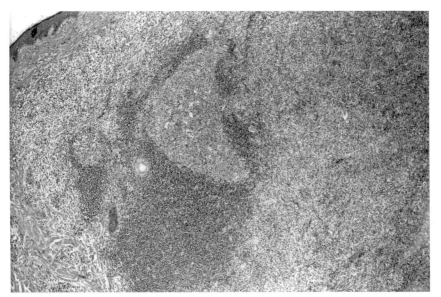

**Fig. 1** Primary cutaneous marginal zone B-cell lymphoma. A residual germinal centre is still present and the mantle zone is expanded.

## FOLLICULAR LYMPHOMA

In follicular lymphoma, the follicles can be regularly or irregularly enlarged, or both. The neoplastic cells are centrocytes and centroblasts and the follicular mantles are usually attenuated or absent (Fig. 2). The neoplastic cells are characteristically CD5-negative but CD10- and/or bcl-6-positive. A very useful finding is the presence of CD10- and/or bcl-6-positive cells in an interfollicular location. A background CD21-positive network is demonstrable.

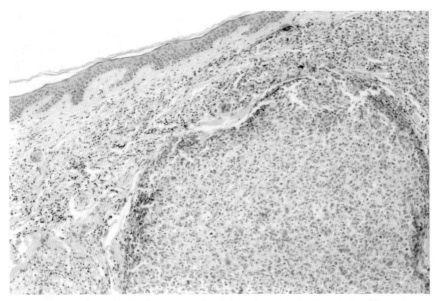

**Fig. 2** Primary cutaneous follicle centre B-cell lymphoma. The neoplastic germinal centre is expanded and the mantle zone is attenuated.

In nodal follicular lymphoma, WHO recommends additional subdivision based on the grade and the percentage of follicular and diffuse areas. This information should be collected in primary follicular cutaneous B-cell lymphoma to facilitate research but its clinical value is currently unproven. Some cutaneous cases conform to the WHO variant of diffuse follicular centre lymphoma.

Several studies have now investigated the frequency of t(14;18) translocation and bcl-2 and bcl-6 molecular abnormalities in primary cutaneous follicular centre lymphoma. The results have been variable and several explanations have been proposed.[23–29] It appears that t(14;18) translocation and bcl-2 re-arrangement is unusual in primary cutaneous follicular centre lymphoma though bcl-2 protein expression may occur on the neoplastic cells. The finding of t(14;18) translocation in follicular cutaneous B-cell lymphoma should trigger a search for possible primary nodal disease.

## DIFFUSE LARGE B-CELL LYMPHOMA

The WHO defines 'large' in this context as exceeding twice the size of a normal lymphocyte; the category includes centroblastic, immunoblastic, T-cell/histiocyte-rich, plasmablastic and anaplastic variants (Fig. 3). The term 'diffuse' and the percentage of large cells required to constitute the entity are not well defined. Many authorities define 'diffuse' by the absence of follicular structures and increasingly by the absence of a follicular dendritic network on CD21 staining. The WHO recommends that when in association with marginal zone lymphoma or follicular lymphoma, diffuse large B-cell lymphoma should be reported as such and not by the term 'high-grade'. The definition of diffuse given by the WHO appears to depend on the presence of solid sheets or confluent areas of large cells.

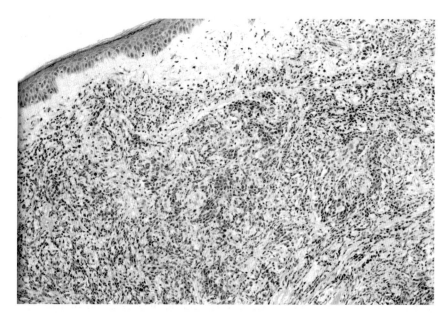

**Fig. 3** Primary cutaneous diffuse large B-cell lymphoma. No follicular structures are present.

The numbers of large cells in the WHO classification vary; it requires more than 15 centroblasts per standard high power field for follicular lymphoma and more than 20 centroblasts per high power field for marginal zone lymphoma. T-cell/histiocyte-rich diffuse large B-cell lymphoma is stated by the WHO to have less than 10% neoplastic cells and immunoblastic diffuse large B-cell lymphoma to have more than 90%. By contrast, other sources have defined diffuse large B-cell lymphoma as a lymphoma in which over 50% of the neoplastic cells are large.[30] The subject of diffuse large B-cell lymphoma has been made complex by the EORTC classification. Many EORTC cases of primary cutaneous follicular centre cell lymphoma occurring on the head and neck constitute examples of diffuse large B-cell lymphoma with a good prognosis. This contrasts with the EORTC category of primary cutaneous large B-cell lymphoma of the leg which is also a diffuse large B-cell lymphoma but has an intermediate prognosis. Not all groups have come to the same prognostic conclusions and so there is considerable debate about diffuse large B-cell lymphoma on the leg.[28,31]

To clarify the situation, a recent European multicentre study has shown that round cell morphology (defined as more than 25% centroblasts or immuno-blasts) was an adverse prognostic factor in all clinical sites whereas multiple lesions were an adverse factor only on the leg.[30] Immunophenotypic and molecular findings in diffuse large B-cell lymphoma are mixed with respect to CD10, bcl-2 and bcl-6 expression and t(14;18) translocation. It is likely that diffuse large B-cell lymphoma constitutes either *de novo* cases or transformed marginal zone or follicular lymphoma. As in nodal lymphoma, gene expression profiling should help to clarify the situation.[13]

## INTRAVASCULAR LARGE B-CELL LYMPHOMA

This rare variant of diffuse large B-cell lymphoma commonly presents in the skin and is characterised by the presence of neoplastic cells in the lumina of small blood vessels and secondary thrombotic sequelae. It is usually systemic at presentation and has a very poor prognosis.

## MANTLE CELL LYMPHOMA

This is a rare disease in the skin and its presence should initiate a search for systemic disease. It is characterised by cyclin D1 and CD5 positivity.

## LYMPHOMATOID GRANULOMATOSIS

Lymphomatoid granulomatosis is an angiocentric and angiodestructive lymphoproliferative disorder which involves extranodal sites. The skin is the commonest extrapulmonary location. The infiltrate is composed of Epstein-Barr virus positive B-cells mixed with greater numbers of reactive T-cells. The disease has a spectrum of clinical aggressiveness which is related to histo-logical grade and proportion of large B-cells. Grade 1 disease is polymorphous with little atypia and few B-cell blasts; clinically, the lesions are indolent and regress spontaneously. Grade 3 disease should be regarded and treated as a variant of diffuse large B-cell lymphoma.

# T-CELL LYMPHOPROLIFERATIVE DISEASES

## MYCOSIS FUNGOIDES AND SÉZARY SYNDROME

Mycosis fungoides is an indolent epidermotropic neoplasm of small-to-medium sized cerebriform T-cells. Clinically, it is characterised by patch, plaque, tumour, erythrodermic and poikilodermatous stages which may overlap. Tumour presentation, in the absence of a preceding stage, should not be diagnosed as mycosis fungoides but as another type of cutaneous T-cell lymphoma. The histological features of mycosis fungoides have been described previously in *Recent Advances in Histopathology* (Fig. 4).[1] Epidermotropism diminishes with increasing stage of disease.[1] A useful diagnostic clue to patch stage is single cell

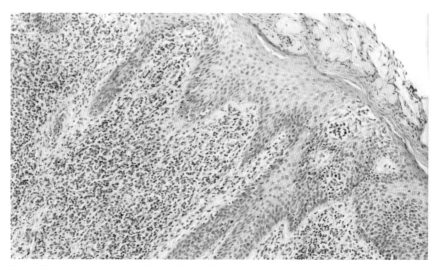

**Fig. 4** Plaque stage mycosis fungoides with Pautrier abscess formation.

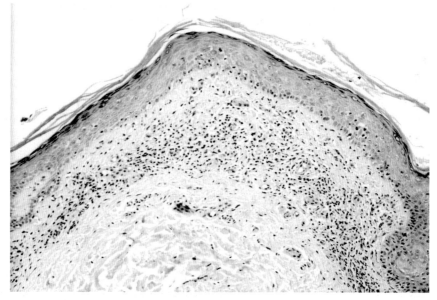

**Fig. 5** Patch stage mycosis fungoides with interface changes and larger atypical cells.

exocytosis with interface changes (Fig. 5). The disease can become biologically high-grade in its later stages: large cell transformation is said to have occurred if large cells constitute more than 25%. The diagnosis of dermatopathic lymphadenopathy in patients with mycosis fungoides can be difficult and genotypic analysis is recommended.

The WHO describes three variants though their inclusion under mycosis fungoides is debatable.

### Pagetoid reticulosis (Woringer-Kolopp disease)

This is a clinically localised and indolent disease. There is pagetoid proliferation of medium-to-large T-cells in the epidermis which also shows acanthosis and sponge-like disaggregation. The phenotypic and genotypic findings are variable.

### Mycosis fungoides-associated follicular mucinosis

This is defined by the presence of medium-to-large T-cells showing folliculotropism rather than epidermotropism with mucinous degeneration of the follicular epithelium. The disease is less responsive to superficial therapy owing to the deeper location of the infiltrate.

### Granulomatous slack skin disease

This is characterised clinically by folds of lax skin that result from a monoclonal T-cell infiltrate. There is elastolysis with elastophagacytosis by multinucleated giant cells.

The criteria for diagnosis of Sézary syndrome defined by the WHO have been overtaken by a more recent report from the International Society for Cutaneous Lymphoma.[32] They consider that Sézary syndrome is the leukaemic phase of erythrodermic cutaneous T-cell lymphoma and distinguish it from erythrodermic mycosis fungoides. Haematological criteria include a Sézary cell count of more than 1000 cells/mm$^3$, a CD4:CD8 ratio greater than 10 and a T-cell monoclone in the peripheral blood.[4] In common with all erythrodermic types of cutaneous T-cell lymphoma, Sézary syndrome has a poor prognosis.

## PRIMARY CUTANEOUS CD30-POSITIVE T-CELL LYMPHOPROLIFERATIVE DISORDERS

These comprise a spectrum of diseases that includes neoplasia (anaplastic large cell lymphoma), T-cell proliferation of uncertain malignant potential (lymphomatoid papulosis) and borderline lesions. The last are disorders in which there is a discrepancy between clinical features and histological appearance, the clinical appearance being the decisive diagnostic criterion. Paradoxically, lymphomatoid papulosis, in this group of the WHO CD30-positive disorders, can even be CD30-negative. The main distinguishing features between this group of diseases are shown in Table 2.

### Primary cutaneous anaplastic large cell lymphoma

A prerequisite for the diagnosis is that systemic anaplastic large cell lymphoma with cutaneous involvement and other types of primary cutaneous lymphoma, especially mycosis fungoides, must be excluded. More than 75% of the large cells must be CD30-positive and the WHO definition is restricted to anaplastic

**Table 2** Primary cutaneous CD30-positive T-cell lymphoproliferative disorders

| Diagnosis | Clinical features | Histopathology |
|---|---|---|
| Lymphoma | Often single nodule/tumour; often persist | Monomorphous (lymphoma) |
| Lymphoma, LYP-like | Often single nodule/tumour; often persist | Polymorphous (LYP-like) |
| LYP types A/B | Multiple, often papules; come and go | Polymorphous (LYP) |
| LYP type C | Multiple, often papules; come and go | Monomorphous (lymphoma-like) |

LYP, lymphomatoid papulosis.

large cells. The latter should comprise at least 30% of the cell population. This is possibly artificial as the diagnostic reproducibility of the assessment of large cell types is questionable. The WHO describes a hallmark anaplastic cell but also describes pleomorphic, round monomorphic, small, signet ring and sarcomatoid cell variants. Nodules or tumours are usually solitary or localised; 10% of patients have nodal involvement and 25% may show partial or complete lesional regression. The cells are usually CD4-positive and are of cytotoxic type. Unlike in systemic anaplastic large cell lymphoma, t(2;5) translocation, ALK-1 protein and EMA expression are usually absent. An interesting histological feature is the frequent association of primary cutaneous anaplastic large cell lymphomas with pseudoepitheliomatous hyperplasia (Fig. 6). The prognosis is favourable in the absence of extracutaneous spread; when possible, chemotherapy should be reserved for this eventuality.

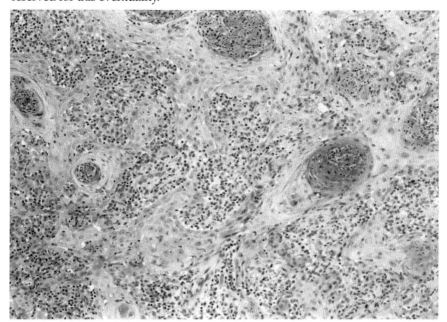

**Fig. 6** Take-away-lesson of the chapter. Pseudoepitheliomatous hyperplasia associated with an underlying primary cutaneous CD30-positive lymphoma. The neoplastic cells can be difficult to find and result in a wrong diagnosis of squamous cell carcinoma.

## Lymphomatoid papulosis

This is a chronic recurring self-healing papulonodular eruption. The T-cells are polyclonal or monoclonal and 10% of cases are preceded by, associated with, or followed by mycosis fungoides, anaplastic large cell lymphoma or Hodgkin's disease. Patients are never cured, but rarely die from their disease. The WHO regards it as proliferation of uncertain malignant potential rather than lymphoma. Different types of lesions have been described histopathologically though these are of no prognostic significance. Type A lesions have many CD30-positive Reed-Sternberg-like cells and numerous mixed inflammatory cells. Type B lesions show predominantly cerebriform cells, with fewer CD30-positive and inflammatory cells (Fig. 7). Mixed type also occur.

## Borderline lesions

Cases that have confluent sheets of CD30-positive anaplastic T-cells which mimic lymphoma histopathologically, and cases with regressing papules that resemble lymphomatoid papulosis clinically are called lymphomatoid papulosis type C. The converse, cases in which there is a solitary skin lymphoma resembling lymphomatoid papulosis histologically, is termed anaplastic lymphoma, lymphomatoid papulosis-like.

## SUBCUTANEOUS PANNICULITIS-LIKE T-CELL LYMPHOMA

Subcutaneous panniculitis-like T-cell lymphoma is a cytotoxic T-cell lymphoma which preferentially infiltrates the subcutis and mimics lobular panniculitis. The adipocytes show characteristic rimming by neoplastic cells which vary in morphology from small and typical to large and atypical. It

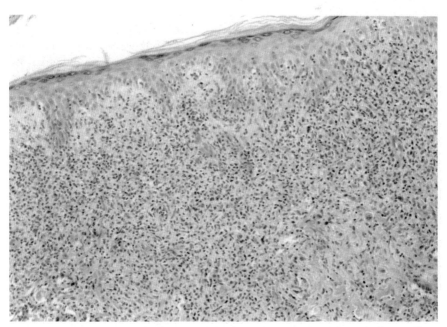

**Fig. 7** Lymphomatoid papulosis. Predominantly type B with atypical cerebriform cells.

conforms to the disease previously called cytophagic histiocytic panniculitis, the name reflecting the predominant histiocytic component with cytophagocytosis manifest by the presence of so-called 'bean-bag' cells. The lymphoma originates from either alpha-beta T-cells which are CD8-positive or gamma-delta T-cells which are CD56-positive and CD4 and CD8 negative. Recent evidence suggests that the latter subgroup has a worst prognosis and a higher incidence of the haemophagocytic syndrome and systemic spread.[33] There is no association with Epstein-Barr virus, but the disease can show similarities with NK/T-cell lymphoma, in terms of CD56 positivity and occasional vascular involvement.[33]

## ANGIOIMMUNOBLASTIC T-CELL LYMPHOMA

Skin manifestations are common and histologically there is a polymorphous infiltrate, blast cells and arborising blood vessels. The blast cells are usually of both T- and Epstein Barr virus positive B-cell lineage mixed with CD21 dendritic cells.

## PERIPHERAL T-CELL LYMPHOMA

The EORTC considers that primary cutaneous CD30-positive large cell lymphoma is a specific clinicopathological category irrespective of its nuclear morphology.[34,35] Collecting data on all CD30 positive types would facilitate further research in this area. It also appears desirable to identify primary cutaneous CD30-negative large cell lymphomas. Large cells should comprise at least 30% of the neoplastic cells. Most CD30-negative large cell lymphomas appear to have an aggressive course; those with more than 80% large pleomorphic cells and immunoblasts have the worst prognosis.[36,37]

The EORTC classification includes a provisional entry of pleomorphic small/medium-sized cutaneous T-cell lymphomas. This is defined by the presence of nodules or tumours with less than 30% of large cells. A recent European study has given further support to the identification of this subtype though the favourable prognosis may be limited to the CD4 rather than CD8 phenotype (Willemze, unpublished presentation). It is uncertain whether the description by Berti et al.[38] of a CD8 cytotoxic medium to large cell lymphoma with an aggressive clinical course is a distinct entity outwith the CD30-negative and CD8-positive considerations already mentioned.

## NK AND NK/T-CELL NEOPLASMS

This group of diseases represents the most significant advance on the REAL and EORTC classifications. Their clinical importance lies in their tendency to have a poor prognosis and respond poorly to treatment. The most useful diagnostic antibody is that against CD56 (neural cell adhesion molecule) though occasionally this can be negative. In a CD56-positive lymphoma, negative surface CD3 and a germline TCR is a good indication of a NK-cell origin. Most cases contain cytoplasmic cytotoxic granules. Because of the immunophenotypic overlap between T- and NK-cells, a source of diagnostic difficulty can be the variable expression by NK-cells of cytoplasmic CD3 and surface CD4, CD8, CD43 and CD45RO. It is important to exclude a non-lymphoid haematological neoplasm as these can be CD56 positive.

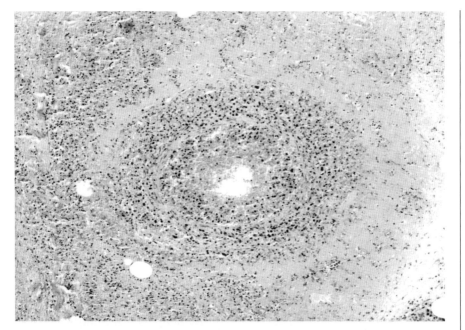

**Fig. 8** Primary cutaneous CD56-positive natural killer lymphoma, nasal type. There is an atypical angiocentric and angiodestructive infiltrate with dermal necrosis. This morphological pattern is indistinguishable from that also seen in lymphomatoid granulomatosis.

Blastic NK-cell lymphoma often presents in the skin as a manifestation of systemic disease.[39] The cells have a lymphoblast-like morphology and consistently express CD4 with other NK-cell markers. There is no association with Epstein-Barr virus.

Extranodal NK/T-cell lymphoma of nasal type is characterised by an angiocentric and angiodestructive infiltrate with coagulative necrosis of the dermis and subcutis (Fig. 8). It is designated NK/T to indicate that it is usually of NK-cell lineage but occasionally has a T-cell origin. The WHO specifies the T-cell type as having an Epstein-Barr virus positive, CD56-negative, cytotoxic T-cell phenotype. The term 'nasal type' highlights that the nasal cavity is the usual site. Cases in the UK have a weaker association with Epstein-Barr virus than elsewhere in the world. Lymphomas apparently originating from CD56-positive NK-like T-cells are currently not recognised by the WHO and should be classified as peripheral T-cell lymphoma.

## Points of best practice

- The diagnosis of cutaneous lymphoma always requires clinicopathological correlation.
- All cases of cutaneous lymphoma must be reviewed by a multidisciplinary team.

## Points of best practice (continued)

- The diagnosis and management of cutaneous lymphoma is a specialised histopathological and dermatological service.

- Cutaneous lymphoma should be classified using the new World Health Organization classification of tumours of haematopoietic and lymphoid tissues.

- When appropriate, histopathology reports of cutaneous lymphoproliferative diseases should contain guidance for clinicians on likely biological behaviour.

- The World Health Organization classification uses a multivariable diagnostic approach and has no one diagnostic gold standard.

- Primary cutaneous CD30-positive T-cell lymphoproliferative disorders are classified using clinical features as the decisive diagnostic criterion.

- Cutaneous lymphoma is rare but one should be vigilant in looking out for it and its variants.

- NK- and NK/T-cell neoplasms are potentially clinically aggressive.

- The World Health Organization classification should be regarded as a road-map, indicating directions for future clinical and scientific research.[40]

## References

1. Slater DN, Lymphoproliferative conditions of the skin. *Recent Adv Histopathol* 1984; **12**: 83–110.
2. Jaffe ES, Harris NL, Stein H, Vardiman JW. *Tumours of Haematopoietic and Lymphoid Tissues, WHO Classification of Tumours*. Lyon: IARC, 2001; 1–351.
3. Willemze R, Kerl H, Sterry W *et al*. EORTC classification for primary cutaneous lymphomas: a proposal from the Cutaneous Lymphoma Study Group of the European Organization for Research and Treatment of Cancer. *Blood* 1997; **90**: 354–371.
4. Russell-Jones R, Whittaker S. T-cell receptor gene analysis in the diagnosis of Sézary syndrome. *J Am Acad Dermatol* 1999; **41**: 254–259.
5. Fraser-Andrews E, Woolford A, Russell-Jones R *et al*. Detection of a peripheral blood T-cell clone is an independent prognostic marker in mycosis fungoides. *J Invest Dermatol* 2000; **114**: 117–121.
6. Whittaker S. Clinical and prognostic significance of molecular studies in cutaneous T-cell lymphoma In: Cerio R. (ed) *Current Topics of Pathology*, vol 94. Berlin: Springer, 2001; 93–101.
7. Child FJ, Woolford AJ, Calonje E *et al*. Molecular analysis of the immunoglobulin heavy gene in the diagnosis of primary cutaneous B-cell lymphoma. *J Invest Dermatol* 2001; **117**: 984–989.
8. Scarisbeck J, Woolford A, Russell-Jones R *et al*. Loss of heterozygosity on 10q and microsatellite instability in advanced stages of primary cutaneous T-cell lymphoma and possible association with homozygous deletion of PTEN. *Blood* 2000; **95**: 2937–2942.
9. McGregor J, Crook T, Fraser-Andrews E *et al*. Spectrum of p53 gene mutations suggests a possible role for ultraviolet radiation in the pathogenesis of advanced cutaneous lymphomas. *J Invest Dermatol* 1999; **112**: 317–321.
10. Gronbaek K, Moller PH, Nedergaard T *et al*. Primary cutaneous B-cell lymphoma: a clinical, histological, phenotypic and genotypic study of 21 cases. *Br J Dermatol* 2000; **142**: 913–923.

11. Child FJ, Scarisbrick JJ, Calonje E *et al*. Inactivation of tumour suppressor genes p15 & p16 in primary cutaneous B-cell lymphoma. *J Invest Dermatol* 2002; **118**: 941–948.
12. Scarisbrick JJ, Woolford AJ, Calonje E *et al*. Frequent abnormalities of the p15 & p16 genes in mycosis fungoides and Sézary syndrome. *J Invest Dermatol* 2002; **118**: 493–499.
13. Alizadeh AA, Elsen MB, Davis ER. Distinct types of diffuse large B-cell lymphoma identified by gene expression profiling. *Nature* 2000; **403**: 503–511.
14. Chan JKC, Banks PM, Cleary ML *et al*. A proposal for classification of lymphoid neoplasms (by the International Lymphoma Study Group). *Histopathology* 1994; **25**: 517–536.
15. Russell-Jones R. Primary cutaneous B-cell lymphoma: how useful is the new European Organization for Research and Treatment of Cancer (EORTC) classification? *Br J Dermatol* 1998; **139**: 945–949.
16. Slater DN. Primary cutaneous B-cell lymphoma: how useful is the new European Organization for Research and Treatment of Cancer (EORTC) classification? *Br J Dermatol* 1999; **141**: 352–353.
17. Jaffe ES, Harris NL, Chan JKC *et al*. Proposed WHO classification of neoplastic diseases of haematopoietic and lymphoid tissues. *Am J Surg Pathol* 1997; **21**: 114–121.
18. Harris NL, Jaffe ES, Diebold J *et al*. The WHO classification of neoplastic disease of the haematopoietic and lymphoid tissues. *Histopathology* 2000; **36**: 69–87.
19. Rooney N, Ramsay A, Norton A *et al*. *Minimum Dataset for the Histopathological Reporting of Lymphoma*. London: The Royal College of Pathologists, 2002; 1–20.
20. Willemze R, Meijer CJLM. EORTC classification for primary cutaneous lymphomas: a comparison with the REAL classification and proposed WHO classification. *Ann Oncol* 2000; **11 (Suppl. 1)**: 511–515.
21. Slater DN. Cutaneous B-cell lymphoproliferative diseases: a centenary celebration classification. *J Pathol* 1994; **172**: 301–305.
22. Slater DN. MALT, SALT: the clue to cutaneous B-cell lymphoproliferative disease. *Br J Dermatol* 1994; **131**: 557–561.
23. de Leval L, Harris NL, Longtine J *et al*. Cutaneous B-cell lymphomas of follicular and marginal zone types. Use of Bcl-6, CD10, Bcl-2 and CD21 in differential diagnosis and classification. *Am J Surg Pathol* 2001; **25**: 732–741.
24. Child FJ, Russell-Jones R, Woolford AJ *et al*. Absence of t(14;18) chromosomal translocation in primary cutaneous B-cell lymphoma. *Br J Dermatol* 2001; **144**: 735–744.
25. Hsi ED, Mirza I, Gascoyne RD. Absence of t(14;18) chromosomal translocation in primary cutaneous B-cell lymphoma. *Br J Dermatol* 2002; **146**: 1110–1111.
26. Child FJ, Russell-Jones R, Calonje E *et al*. Absence of t(14;18) chromosomal translocation in primary cutaneous B-cell lymphoma. *Br J Dermatol* 2001; **146**: 1111–1112.
27. Franco R, Fernandez-Vazquez A, Rodriguez-Peralto JL *et al*. Cutaneous follicular B-cell lymphoma. Description of a series of 18 cases. *Am J Surg Pathol* 2001; **25**: 875–883.
28. Yang B, Tubbs RR, Finn W *et al*. Clinicopathological assessment of primary cutaneous B-cell lymphoma with immunophenotypic and molecular genetic characterisation. *Am J Surg Pathol* 2000: **24**: 694–702.
29. Goodlad JR, Krajewski AS, Batstone PJ *et al*. Primary cutaneous follicular lymphoma. A clinicopathologic and molecular study of 16 cases in support of a distinct entity. *Am J Surg Pathol* 2002; **26**: 733–741.
30. Grange F, Bekkenk MW, Wechsler J *et al*. Prognostic factors in primary cutaneous large B-cell lymphomas; a European multicentre study. *J Clin Oncol* 2001; **19**: 3602–3610.
31. Fernandez-Vazquez A, Rodriquez-Peralto JL, Martinez MA *et al*. Primary cutaneous large B-cell lymphoma. The relation between morphology, clinical presentation, immunohistochemical markers and survival. *Am J Surg Pathol* 2001; **25**: 307–315.
32. Vonderheid EC, Bernengo MG, Burg G *et al*. Update on erythrodermic cutaneous T-cell lymphoma: report of the International Society for Cutaneous Lymphoma. *J Am Acad Dermatol* 2002; **46**: 95–106.
33. Hoque SR, Child FJ, Whittaker SJ *et al*. Subcutaneous panniculitis-like T-cell lymphoma: a clinicopathological, immunophenotypic and molecular analysis of 6 patients. *Br J Dermatol* 2003; **148**: 516–525.
34. Beljaards RC, Kaudewitz P, Berti E *et al*. Primary cutaneous CD30 positive large cell lymphoma: definition of a new type of cutaneous lymphoma with a favourable prognosis. A European multicentre study on 47 cases. *Cancer* 1993; **71**: 2097–2120.

35. Paulli M, Berti E, Rosso R *et al*. CD30/Ki-1 positive lymphoproliferative disorders of the skin. Clinicopathologic correlation and statistical analysis of 86 cases. A multicentre study from the EORTC cutaneous lymphoma study group *J Clin Oncol* 1996; **13**: 1343–1362.

36. Beljaards RC, Meijer CJLM, Scheffer E *et al*. Prognostic significance of CD30/Ki-I/Ber-H2 expression of primary cutaneous large-cell lymphomas of T-cell origin. A clinicopathologic and immunohistochemical study in 20 patients. *Am J Pathol* 1989; **135**: 1169–1182.

37. Beljaards RC, Meijer CJLM, van der Putte SCJ *et al*. Primary cutaneous T-cell lymphomas. Clinicopathological features of prognostic parameters of 35 cases other than mycosis fungoides and CD30-positive large cell lymphoma. *J Pathol* 1994; **172**: 53–65.

38. Berti E, Tomasini D, Vermeer MH *et al*. Primary cutaneous CD8-positive epidermotropic cytotoxic T-cell lymphoma. *Am J Pathol* 1999; **155**: 483–492.

39. Child FJ, Mitchell TJ, Whittaker SJ *et al*. Blastic natural killer and extranodal natural killer-like T-cell lymphoma presenting in the skin: report of 6 cases from the UK. *Br J Dermatol* 2003; **148**: 507–515.

40. Sander CA, Flaig MJ, Jaffe ES. Cutaneous manifestations of lymphoma: a clinical guide based on the WHO classification. *Clin Lymphoma* 2001; **2**: 86–100.

*R.L. Attanoos   A.R. Gibbs*

**5**

# Asbestos-related neoplasia

Asbestos exposure constitutes a major health hazard in all industrialised countries and about 1 in 5 people world-wide are exposed to asbestos during their lifetime. Almost all exposures are occupational but some may be through domestic (para-occupational), neighbourhood or environmental (ambient) sources. The total cancer burden of asbestos in Western industrialised countries has been calculated to be about 30,000 asbestos-related cancers per year.[1]

There is unavoidable daily low level background exposure to asbestos within and outside buildings regardless of occupation; past occupational exposures to asbestos were several orders of magnitude higher than general environmental exposures. There is no evidence to indicate that general background exposures cause disease. In the evaluation of a potential asbestos-related disease any use of asbestos body or asbestos fibre counts should take account of the background ranges determined by the laboratory carrying out the test. Over the past decade there has been a change in the type of occupation prone to asbestos-related diseases. Up to the 1980s in industrialised countries, most cases resulted from asbestos exposures in the asbestos products, insulation, and shipyard industries: nowadays, cases (particularly mesotheliomas) occur in the construction and power-generating industries and are also seen in electricians and plumbers.

Assessment of exposure to asbestos can be difficult in people unless they have been occupationally exposed in well-recognised situations as the relevant exposures may have been several decades before the development of the asbestos-related disease and exposures might have been indirect. The histopathologist can provide a more objective means of verifying exposure by the finding of asbestos bodies or by submitting lung tissue for mineral fibre analysis.

**R.L. Attanoos** BSc MBBS FRCPath
Consultant Pathologist, Department of Pathology, Llandough Hospital, Cardiff and Vale NHS Trust, Penarth, South Glamorgan CF64 2XX, UK

**Dr A.R. Gibbs** TD MB ChB FRCPath
Consultant Pathologist, Department of Histopathology, Llandough Hospital, Cardiff and Vale NHS Trust, Penarth, South Glamorgan CF64 2XX, UK. Tel: +44 29 2071 5283; Fax: +44 29 2071 2979
(for correspondence)

There are two major groups of asbestos fibres, the distinction being important because there is a much lower potential for induction of disease by chrysotile than the amphiboles as the lung clears chrysotile much more efficiently. The serpentine group contains one type of asbestos, chrysotile (white), the most widely used commercial form; the amphibole group includes several types including the commercial forms crocidolite (blue) and amosite (brown) and the non-commercial forms tremolite, anthophyllite and actinolite.

## MALIGNANT MESOTHELIOMA

Malignant mesothelioma used to be a rare tumour. Since 1960 when exposure to crocidolite was recognised as a cause of mesothelioma the neoplasm has increased in incidence and most general histopathologists will see a case from time-to-time in their practice. In industrialised countries, the annual incidence of mesothelioma is 14–30 cases per million adults and in the UK the annual incidence has risen from 154 cases in 1968 to 1330 in 1997; the increase is greater in males (7-fold) than in females (4-fold).[2] The background, spontaneous rate of mesothelioma has been estimated at 1–2 per million per year.

### AETIOLOGY

The strongest aetiological link recognised so far has been exposure to asbestos, particularly the amphibole forms, and the incidence of mesothelioma in most countries parallels the previous use of amphibole asbestos. In the UK, it has been estimated that 80–90% of mesotheliomas in men and about 60% in women were caused by exposure to asbestos. Exposures to asbestos in women are more commonly through the domestic than the direct occupational route. A recent study found that the relative risks for the development of mesothelioma for the various different fibre types is: 1 (chrysotile), 100 (amosite), and 500 (crocidolite).[3] Latency in regard to asbestos-related mesothelioma is measured from first exposure to asbestos to death from mesothelioma. A review of 1690 cases of mesothelioma found that 99% had a latent period of more than 15 years; 96% had a latent period of at least 20 years with a median of 32 years.[4]

Other potential aetiological agents include: (i) exposure to a non-asbestos fibre called erionite which is present in the Cappadocian region of Turkey; (ii) therapeutic radiation for tumours such as Wilms' tumour and lymphoma; (iii) thorium dioxide (thorotrast) exposure; and (iv) chronic irritation of serosal surfaces. Recently, there has been much interest in simian virus 40, the protein sequences of which have been identified in tissue specimens of mesotheliomas from several countries. This virus contaminated poliomyelitis and other vaccines in the 1950s and early 1960s. The virus is oncogenic, can induce mesothelioma in animals and can interact with the tumour suppressor gene products p53 and pRb so may have a role in the pathogenesis of mesothelioma.[5,6]

### CLINICAL FEATURES

More than 90% of malignant mesotheliomas are primary pleural in origin; 6–10% are of peritoneal origin. *Bona fide* cases of malignant mesothelioma of the

**Table 1** Light microscopic patterns of malignant mesothelioma

| Epithelioid | Mixed | Sarcomatoid |
|---|---|---|
| Tubulopapillary | Any combination | Cellular storiform |
| Clear cell | | Desmoplastic |
| Adenomatoid | | Leiomyoid |
| Solid | | Chondroid |
| Small cell | | Osseous |
| Pleomorphic | | Lymphohistiocytoid |
| Mucin-positive | | |
| Deciduoid | | |

pericardium, tunica vaginalis of the testis and ovary are very rare. The clinical presentation is often non-specific with lassitude, anorexia, weight loss or gain, pleuritic or abdominal pain and signs of an associated effusion. Rarely mesotheliomas can present with metastases. The clinical course is progressive and relentless with no curative treatment and the patient dies on average 9–12 months from diagnosis. Few cases survive more than 2 years after diagnosis. There is intensive research into new modalities of treatment and clinical trials of various chemotherapeutic agents which may alter the prognosis in the near future.

## DIAGNOSTIC CONSIDERATIONS

The diagnosis of malignant mesothelioma is facilitated by a multidisciplinary approach which assimilates clinical, radiological and pathological information. In typical cases of malignant mesothelioma, diffuse serosal growth with minimal visceral invasion is common. Localised malignant mesothelioma is very rare. Non-mesothelial tumours (mostly carcinomas) can diffusely involve the visceral and parietal pleura and peritoneum; clinically, radiologically and macroscopically they mimic malignant mesothelioma. These so-called 'pseudomesotheliomas' are commonly adenocarcinomas; sarcoma, lymphoma, thymic epithelial tumours, and metastatic neoplasms may also mimic mesothelioma clinically and on microscopy.

The light microscopic diagnosis of malignant mesothelioma is problematic because of its morphological diversity and capacity to mimic histogenetically diverse neoplasms and reactive conditions. The World Health Organization's classification for lung and pleural tumours recognises three basic subtypes of malignant mesothelioma – epithelioid, biphasic and sarcomatoid. This is of prognostic significance as epithelioid forms have a better prognosis. In our view this is a gross oversimplification and several architectural patterns have been described within each of the subtypes (Table 1). Whilst not clinically important, an awareness of these patterns is important in recognition of the tumour.

## SEROSAL BIOPSY INTERPRETATION

Closed pleural needle biopsies often produce specimens 0.3–0.5 cm long which have a low diagnostic yield in suspected cases of malignant mesothelioma. In our series of 53 pleural biopsies, a definitive diagnosis of malignant

**Table 2** Serosal biopsy interpretation

| |
|---|
| Is the biopsy adequate? |
| Is there evidence of neoplasia? |
|        Primary or secondary (histogenetic type)? |
| Reactive changes – nil suspicious |
| Are there worrying features that require follow-up or re-biopsy? |

mesothelioma could be made in 25% of closed and 90% of open thoracoscopic pleural biopsy specimens.[7] Serosal biopsy interpretation requires systematic assessment (Table 2). An adequate specimen has mesothelium with subjacent fibroconnective tissue, though metastatic tumour can be identified with the aid of immunohistochemistry in the absence of mesothelium.

The diagnostic distinction between a reactive mesothelial proliferation and malignant mesothelioma is particularly problematic because reactive mesothelial hyperplasia can be very cellular, mitotically active, and cytologically atypical, and can form 'pseudo-invasive' islands of entrapped mesothelial cells in areas of organising pleuritis. Conversely, malignant mesothelioma can be cytologically bland. Important discriminating factors between mesothelial hyperplasia and malignant mesothelioma are shown in Table 3. For spindle cell proliferations, the distinction between desmoplastic malignant mesothelioma and fibrous pleuritis is even more difficult. In our study, closed pleural biopsy diagnosis of sarcomatoid malignant mesothelioma was 12% when present. Frank invasion and bland necrosis are regarded as the two most significant discriminating diagnostic features.

Our favoured immunohistochemical panel for the differential diagnosis of reactive mesothelial hyperplasia versus epithelioid mesothelioma is epithelial membrane antigen (EMA), p53 and desmin which cover benign and malignant mesothelial proliferations. EMA and p53 are preferentially expressed on the neoplastic mesothelial cell membrane and nucleus, respectively, and desmin is preferentially expressed in benign mesothelial cell cytoplasm. These markers will not distinguish reactive from neoplastic spindle cell proliferations; p53 staining is very dependent on fixation and is positive in only half of malignant mesotheliomas.

The recognition of metastatic tumour in a serosal biopsy has been greatly assisted by the developments in immunohistochemistry. Many publications

**Table 3** Discriminant markers in reactive and neoplastic mesothelium

| Diagnostic factors | Malignant mesothelioma | Mesothelial hyperplasia |
|---|---|---|
| Frank invasion | + (fat/viscera) | – (beware entrapment) |
| Cell proliferation | No polarity | Polarity to surface |
| Necrosis | Bland ± | Absent (except TB & RA) |
| EMA | + (membrane) | Focal + or – |
| p53 | + (nuclear) | – |
| Desmin | –/focal + | + |

TB, tuberculosis; RA, rheumatoid arthritis.

have addressed the issue of discriminating pleural mesothelioma from pulmonary adenocarcinoma. More recently, publications have addressed the impact of new specific mesothelial markers in facilitating diagnosis. The diagnostic panel should include two or more mesothelial and two or more epithelial markers.

## MESOTHELIAL MARKERS

Broad spectrum cytokeratin (AE1/3) is a sensitive but non-specific marker for malignant mesothelioma. It has application in distinguishing sarcomatoid mesothelioma from most sarcomas and from solitary fibrous tumour. About 15% of sarcomatous mesotheliomas are cytokeratin-negative: synovial sarcoma and leiomyosarcoma can be cytokeratin-positive.

Cytokeratin 5/6 is a useful marker for epithelioid mesothelioma but has low specificity (30%) for sarcomatoid mesothelioma. It is frequently expressed in squamous carcinoma, transitional cell carcinoma and thymic epithelial tumours which can mimic solid epithelioid and lymphohistiocytoid forms of malignant mesothelioma.

Calretinin is the most consistently reliable mesothelial marker with high specificity and sensitivity for epithelioid mesothelioma and 40% specificity for sarcomatoid mesothelioma. Care should be exercised in its interpretation – only nuclear expression is considered to be specific. Cases of renal cell carcinoma, intestinal adenocarcinoma and synovial sarcoma have been found to stain positively for calretinin.

Thrombomodulin is expressed by mesothelium, endothelium, squamous and transitional epithelium, syncytiotrophoblast and synovium. Neoplasms derived from these tissues also express thrombomodulin. Thrombomodulin is positive in half of mesotheliomas in most series and there is little expression in sarcomatoid forms.

The use of N-cadherin and Wilms' tumour susceptibility gene-1 in the differential diagnosis requires more investigation. HBME-1 and CD44H have low specificity and sensitivity and are difficult to interpret; we do not advocate their use. Our preferred epithelial markers are monoclonal carcino-embryonic antigen (CEA), BerEP4 and MOC-31. Thyroid transcription factor-1 (TTF-1) is also useful in the identification of a primary pulmonary neoplasm and is negative in malignant mesothelioma.

Suspicious features of the epithelioid subtype of malignant mesothelioma in biopsies include papillary mesothelial structures, marked atypia, abnormal mitotic features, and immunophenotypically florid EMA or p53 expression (irrespective of cytology). Suspicious features of the sarcomatoid subtype of malignant mesothelioma include high cellularity, cellular disarray, and cytological atypia. In small biopsies, the presence of any of these suspicious features, particularly in light of clinical suspicion, justify a report of 'atypical mesothelial proliferation' and a request for a repeat biopsy, preferably obtained thoracoscopically or by thoracotomy. A history of asbestos exposure is irrelevant to the diagnostic decision-making process.

At post mortem examination, the role of the pathologist in suspected cases of malignant mesothelioma is to determine the tumour diagnosis, determine the aetiology if possible, and assess concomitant disease which might have caused death or had an impact on life expectancy. Post mortem handling of malignant mesothelioma cases has previously been described in detail.[8]

Mineral analysis by electron microscopy for determination of asbestos fibre burden is recommended if: (i) the asbestos exposure history is unclear or suggests mixed or complex dust exposure; no other asbestos-related conditions are identified; and (iii) asbestos bodies are absent in lung sections.[9]

---

## Points of best practice

- About 80–90% of mesotheliomas occur in men with more than 20 years' latency after exposure to asbestos.

- Malignant mesothelioma can follow relatively low level, intermittent or brief exposures to asbestos.

- Over 99% have a diffuse serosal growth pattern (though this is not pathognomonic).

- Morphologically, it has diverse features and mimics reactive conditions and epithelioid and sarcomatous neoplasms.

- Useful mesothelial markers are broad spectrum cytokeratin, calretinin and cytokeratin 5/6.

- Useful epithelial markers include CEA, CD15, BerEP4, MOC31 and TTF-1.

- EMA, p53 and desmin are useful in distinguishing reactive from neoplastic mesothelial proliferations.

---

## ASBESTOS-RELATED LUNG CANCER

The association between lung cancer and asbestos was made in the 1930s but established in 1955 in an epidemiological mortality study of asbestos workers.[10]

### HISTOLOGICAL TYPE

Some studies report adenocarcinoma as the most common histological subtype but others indicate that all four major histological types of lung cancer occur in proportions little different from control cases.[11] In the US, it has been estimated that more than half of the 9000–10,000 men and 900–1900 women developing occupational-related lung cancer annually have had previous asbestos exposure.[12] Histological type has no value in proving or disproving a relation to asbestos.

### ANATOMICAL SITE

No major differences have been found in the proportion of peripheral versus central cancers in patients who have been exposed to asbestos.[11] Several studies have recorded a predominance of lower lobe carcinoma in asbestos-exposed people with an upper lobe to lower lobe ratio of about 1:2.

## ASBESTOS EXPOSED COHORTS

Lung cancer risk in asbestos workers varies with industrial process. It is high in insulators, intermediate in textile workers and low in friction-product workers and asbestos cement manufacturers.

## ASBESTOS FIBRE TYPE

Lung cancer risk varies with fibre type. There are consistently higher rates in occupational cohorts exposed to amphibole than to chrysotile.

## LUNG CANCER, TOBACCO SMOKE AND ASBESTOS

Published studies of tobacco consumption and asbestos show a synergism which ranges from a more-than-additive to a supra-multiplicative effect. Recently, Liddell[13] has suggested that by statistical modelling a less than multiplicative interaction between tobacco smoke and asbestos exists in increasing lung cancer risk. Importantly, non-smokers have a relative risk of lung cancer from asbestos exposure that is about twice as high as the relative risk for smokers. The absolute risk of lung cancer is, of course substantially less in non-smokers than in smokers.

It was previously believed that cessation of long-term smoking results in normalisation of lung cancer risk; more recent data indicate that while smoking cessation is beneficial at any age, risk reduction is far less than complete. For example, smoking cessation for 50 years results in a 5% excess lung cancer risk in people aged 75–80 years. This is important when considering the synergism between smoking in ex-smokers and asbestos in medicolegal cases.

## PATHOGENESIS

Tobacco smoke contains many carcinogens which stimulate mutations in bronchial epithelial cells and cause oncogenic alterations. The synergistic mechanisms between asbestos and tobacco in increasing lung cancer risk include the possibility of tobacco carcinogen adsorption onto asbestos fibres facilitating cellular uptake and decreased fibre clearance in smokers. Chronic inflammation in response to asbestos inhalation leads to epithelial proliferation and increased risk of mutagenesis.[14] Pulmonary fibrosis may compromise the host's capacity to undertake cellular reparative change. The synergism observed with asbestos and tobacco for bronchial carcinoma is a feature of malignant mesotheliomas, so for different target cells the mechanisms of action of asbestos must vary.

## ASBESTOS, ASBESTOSIS AND LUNG CANCER: CONTROVERSIES

The literature is somewhat contradictory and all published studies have inherent design flaws. Prospective cohort mortality studies in which asbestos exposures in workers are well-defined are more useful in addressing questions on causation when compared to retrospective, case-referent studies. Epidemiological studies are limited in demonstrating a low level effect in a high incidence lesion such as lung cancer. Case-referent studies and post mortem studies are often criticised for selection bias of cases or controls or both. Pathological and mineralogical studies are often criticised for lack of standardisation of terminology or laboratory technique.

## Asbestosis: problems with diagnosis

The diagnosis of all interstitial lung disease should be based on the summation of clinical, radiological and pathological information. There is much clinical and radiological overlap among different forms of diffuse interstitial fibrosis (including asbestosis) that such factors cannot be reliably used to distinguish the different conditions. The pathological diagnosis of asbestosis represents the most specific means of confirming diagnosis. It is worth remembering that asbestosis is often a symmetric process with lower lobe and subpleural accentuation.

Asbestosis is defined as diffuse interstitial fibrosis caused by asbestos. The two essential elements for the light microscopic diagnosis are interstitial fibrosis and asbestos bodies. The interpretation of the term 'diffuse' is problematic. True diffuse interstitial fibrotic changes occur only when there is fibrotic bridging between respiratory bronchioles – grade 3 fibrosis. This would correlate to radiologically detectable changes on chest X-ray, clinically apparent symptomatology and restrictive lung function defects. If 'diffuse interstitial fibrosis' is interpreted in this way there will be clinical evidence of asbestosis. However, asbestosis is a clinically slowly progressive condition which begins multifocally around respiratory bronchioles causing changes which are subclinical and subradiological. The minimal diagnostic criteria as determined by CAP–NIOSH for asbestosis requires 'fibrosis around respiratory bronchioles with accumulations of asbestos bodies'. Mild peribronchiolar fibrosis constitutes grade 1 fibrosis; this is not specific to asbestosis and can be identified in many old people, particularly smokers, and in association with other mineral and organic dusts. In our opinion, if the deceased was a current or ex-smoker, then the attribution of peribronchiolar fibrosis to asbestos should be made cautiously and is reliant on the demonstration of extensive multifocal and lower lobe accentuated changes. Conversely, a diagnosis of asbestosis should not be made in smokers or ex-smokers with predominant upper lobe disease.

The proportion of asbestos fibres which become coated to form asbestos bodies varies with fibre type and host immune factors. Amphiboles (especially amosite) form asbestos bodies more readily than chrysotile. In general, there is a loose correlation between asbestos body count and the severity of asbestosis. The number of asbestos bodies required to diagnose asbestosis has not been standardised and varies from the identification of 1–2 or more per $cm^2$. Pseudo-asbestos bodies are ferruginous bodies forming on non-asbestos fibres such as iron, elastin, sheet silicates, erionite or man-made mineral fibres (glasswool, rockwool) which are sometimes incorrectly identified as asbestos bodies.

Very rarely, patients with asbestosis have interstitial fibrosis with few or no asbestos bodies because they do not coat asbestos fibres. Mineral fibre analysis demonstrates a relatively high asbestos fibre burden is such cases and this should be within the range recorded for established cases of asbestosis for the laboratory. Asbestos fibre burdens vary according to the extent (grade) of fibrosis and the ranges and median values for grade 1 fibrosis will be very different from those for grade 3/4 fibrosis.

There is considerable controversy over whether asbestos *per se* or asbestosis increases lung cancer. Presently medical opinion is divided into three groups: (i) any asbestos exposure increases the risk of lung cancer; (ii) the risk of lung cancer is increased only when exposure is sufficient to produce asbestosis (even in the absence of asbestosis itself); and (iii) the risk of lung cancer is increased only when asbestosis is present.

## FIBROSIS–CANCER HYPOTHESIS

Numerous studies have shown that lung cancer risk is increased in the presence of clinical asbestosis, constituting 30–50% of deaths in some series. In general, medical opinion is that lung cancer risk is increased in the presence of asbestosis. The proponents of the fibrosis–cancer hypothesis advocate that it is only in the presence of asbestos-induced lung fibrosis that lung cancer risk is increased – that is, asbestos fibres do not confer an increased risk of lung cancer unless fibrosis is present. They justify this position by the following observations:

- Diffuse interstitial fibrosis of non-asbestos aetiology is also associated with increased risk of lung cancer

- Epidemiological studies show a link between asbestosis and lung cancer and not asbestos exposure *per se*

- In animal inhalation studies, lung cancers develop in only those animals with asbestosis.

The pathogenetic mechanism advocated by many supporters of the fibrosis–cancer hypothesis is that following inhalation, partial macrophage ingestion of asbestos fibres occurs. Subsequent release of lymphokines, growth factors, proteolytic enzymes and free radicals occurs and these soluble factors have the capacity to produce fibrosis as well as eventually being genotoxic and causing lung cancer. Most advocates of the fibrosis–cancer hypothesis do not suggest that the lung cancer develops as a direct consequence of local tissue fibrosis (scar cancer).

It should be highlighted that many of the epidemiological cohort mortality studies demonstrating increased lung cancer risk in the presence of asbestosis were based on radiologically detectable changes; at a pathological level this approximates to grade 3 fibrosis. It is not clear that the risk of asbestos-related lung cancer is increased in the subclinical levels of grades 1 to 2 fibrosis. The publications supporting this hypothesis are given in Table 4.

## FIBRE BURDEN HYPOTHESIS

On the assumption of a linear dose-response, the proponents of the fibre burden hypothesis maintain that any asbestos exposure increases the risk of lung cancer. The main exponents of this view convened an International Expert Meeting in Helsinki in 1997 and they cited the following in justification:[19]

- *In vitro* studies indicate that asbestos can induce transformation in cells along a gradient (mesothelial > bronchial epithelial > fibroblasts). This implies that, hypothetically, carcinogenicity and fibrogenicity are separate processes

- Lung cancer incidence in asbestos-exposed regions does not correlate with incidence of asbestosis

- Lung cancer risk is raised in the absence of radiologically detectable changes on chest X-ray

- Epidemiological studies identify the effect of high exposure seen in asbestosis and lung cancer but do not indicate that at lower exposure there is no increased lung cancer risk

- Lung cancer risk has been correlated to increased fibre burden independent of fibrosis and smoking.

The publications supporting the fibre – burden hypothesis are summarised in Table 5.

In one mineral analytical study undertaken by scanning electron microscopy the authors suggested that a retained lung mineral fibre content of 5 million

**Table 4** Key publications for fibrosis–cancer link hypothesis

| Authors | Study design | Results and comments |
|---|---|---|
| Doll (1955)[10] | Cohort mortality of textile workers with high SMR exposures | Increased lung cancer only in men with asbestosis |
| Bohlig *et al.* (1960)[15] | Retrospective | Lung cancer: 8/1000 with severe asbestosis; 1/1000 minimal asbestosis and 0.4 /1000 no fibrosis. The latter equates to the background incidence of lung cancer in non-asbestos exposed population |
| Sluis–Kremer & Bezuidenhout (1989)[16] | Necropsy study of 339 amphibole miners | Lung cancer SMR increased (up to almost 6-fold) in the presence of moderate/severe asbestosis but not without. Smoking, age and degree of fibrosis correlated with lung cancer risk Comment: only 36.7% of workforce (all white) studied – selection bias. Pathology: non- standard terminology used |
| Weiss (1990)[17] | Meta-analysis of 38 cohorts. Correlated 7 cohorts | Where there were no deaths from asbestosis, lung cancer SMRs were 100. Other studies which showed prominent asbestosis showed excess lung cancer risk |
| Hughes & Weill (1991)[18] | Prospective mortality of 839 asbestos cement workers | Lung cancer SMR increased (4-fold) only in those with radiologically detectable irregular opacities (*i.e.* radiological evidence of asbestosis ILO >1/0). Comment: cohort size too small to identify all lung cancers |

**Table 5** Key publications for asbestos increases risk of lung cancer (fibre burden link)

**Authors:** De Vos Irvine *et al.* (1993)[20]

*Study design:* Questionnaire

*Results and comments:* Report argues that lung cancer in Western Scotland is not related to reported incidence of cases of asbestosis suggesting that fibrosis is not a prerequisite to lung cancer in asbestos exposure individuals. Comment: the authors used incidence of known chronic obstructive pulmonary disease as a surrogate marker of smoking, malignant mesothelioma as a marker of asbestos exposure and reported asbestosis claims to assess rates of asbestosis. The surrogate markers are too non-specific and asbestosis rates are often underestimated. There is no reference to the presence/absence of asbestosis in the study groups

**Authors:** Karjalainen *et al.* (1994)[21]

*Study design:* Fibre analysis (SEM) of 113 lung cancers and comparison to laboratory controls

*Results and comments:* Odds ratio after adjusting for smoking, age and fibrosis revealed a 2-fold increase in lung cancer was associated with retained asbestos fibre levels above 2 million (> 5 μm)/g dry lung tissue or 5 million (> 1 μm)/g dry lung tissue. In a medicolegal setting a 2-fold increase in risk constitutes a significant causal effect. Comment: mineral analysis results are dependent on laboratory technique and the absolute figures only applies to the Finnish laboratory.

**Authors:** Wilkinson *et al.* (1995)[22]

*Study design:* Case-referent of 271 lung cancer patients and 678 referents with occupations detailed and CXR reviewed for irregular opacities

*Results and comments:* Odds ratio 2.3 for fibrosis (ILO > 1/0) and 1.56 for no fibrosis (ILO < 0/1). Criticisms include potential confounding by other mineral dusts, unusual controls (persons with cardiorespiratory disease in East London), sub-radiological degrees of asbestosis may have been present (grades 1 & 2) and so the results in no way contradict the view that fibrosis in a subcohort of persons increases risk of lung cancer. The odds ratio between cases and referents was higher in 'probable asbestos group' compared to 'definite asbestos exposed group' suggesting methodological design flaws

amphibole asbestos fibres per gram of dry lung was associated with a 2-fold increase in lung cancer risk.[21] However, data from transmission electron microscopy do not support the findings proposed by the Helsinki meeting.[19] Analysis of 189 Devonport dockyard workers with a known standardised mortality ratio for lung cancer of 107 (much less than a doubling of risk) demonstrated a median amphibole content of 18 million fibres per gram of dry lung.[23] In our opinion, this raises concerns about the figure of 5 million amphibole asbestos fibres per gram of dry lung equating to a doubling of risk for lung cancer.

## LARYNGEAL CANCER

Laryngeal cancer is an uncommon malignancy and can be divided into three types – glottic, supraglottic and subglottic – which have different mortality

## Points for best practice

- Animal experiments, epidemiological cohort studies on asbestos exposed workers, radiological and pathological evidence indicate that lung cancer risk is increased in the presence of asbestosis.

- There is a synergistic link between asbestos exposure and tobacco smoking in increasing the risk of lung cancer. The synergism is dependent on cumulative asbestos exposure and tobacco pack-years.

- The histological type and anatomical site of lung cancer are not useful in distinguishing smoking from asbestos-related neoplasms.

- Lung cancer risk may or may not be materially increased in the absence of lung fibrosis (asbestosis). The fibre burden hypothesis (that any asbestos exposure increases lung cancer risk) requires further substantiation.

- Pleural lesions in asbestos-exposed persons are very common, occur with low-dose exposures to asbestos and do not confer an increased risk of lung cancer. In the UK, financial compensation for asbestos-related lung cancer is granted when the patient has asbestosis or asbestos-related diffuse pleural fibrosis, or both, though there is no supportive evidence indicating a causal link with the latter.

- Mineral fibre analysis results vary considerably among laboratories and, as different technical methodologies are used, they are applicable only to the laboratory. Conclusions reached in the Helsinki criteria that asbestos fibre burdens are associated with a 2-fold increased risk of lung cancer are fundamentally flawed. Each laboratory is required to define the range levels for each asbestos-related pathology.

rates and which may have different risk factors. When trying to assess the risk of this cancer from exposure to asbestos major confounding factors have to be allowed for, particularly tobacco and alcohol. Social class, diet and temporal changes may also play a part.

Tobacco and alcohol are established factors for laryngeal cancer. Muscat and Wynder[24] provided the following ratios for relative risk: cigarette smokers to non-smokers, 14:1; alcohol consumption > 20 units per day, 7:1.

There have been several cohort studies which have given mortality rates for laryngeal cancer in relation to asbestos exposure and about half have suggested a greater risk. These studies have been in cohorts with high alcohol and tobacco usage and it is probable that the small excess of cases would disappear if these two confounding factors were controlled for. There seems to be no reliable evidence that asbestos exposure is a cause of laryngeal cancer.[2] Case control studies also show no good evidence of an excess risk for laryngeal cancer from asbestos exposure.[25]

## STOMACH AND COLORECTAL CANCER

Colorectal cancer is the second most frequent cause of cancer-related deaths in males. The major risk factors implicated in its causation have been genetic influences and diet. Other factors have been postulated including alcohol and tobacco consumption.

Initially, a link between asbestos exposure and colorectal cancer was suggested by epidemiological studies of insulation workers. Epidemiological studies of this issue have been conflicting, have lacked consistency and have not been well controlled for confounding factors. Weiss[17] reviewed 21 asbestos-exposed cohort studies in which standardised morbidity or mortality ratios were provided. He found that the summary standardised mortality or morbidity ratio for all the cohorts was 0.97 ($P > 0.05$) and there was no dose-response relation in the two studies which provided such data. Epidemiological and animal studies have failed to show any association between colorectal cancer and asbestos ingestion.

After an initial report suggesting a link between asbestos exposure and stomach cancer, there have been many cohort studies which have not shown an increased risk. There is a strong difference in relative risk between social classes for stomach cancer – about 1:3 between classes 1 and 5 in the UK. This is a strong confounder when examining the link between asbestos exposure and stomach cancer. A recent study by Kang et al.[26] examined death certificates from 4,934,566 decedents with information on occupation and industry from 28 states from 1979–1990 and identified occupations with potentially high numbers of workers exposed to asbestos from raised proportionate mortality ratios for mesothelioma. In the 12 occupations with elevated proportionate mortality ratios for mesothelioma, 15,524 cases of gastrointestinal cancer were found giving overall raised ratios for oesophageal, gastric and colorectal cancer. Kang's group concluded that there was an association between asbestos exposure and some gastrointestinal cancer, but the link was small. This conclusion appears difficult to justify as the proportionate mortality ratios were not consistently raised for gastrointestinal cancer for each occupational group, in particular insulation workers where asbestos exposures are amongst the highest. Death certificate information provides very limited information about asbestos exposure and does not allow for controlling of other confounding factors such as diet, exercise, alcohol and tobacco consumption and socio-economic status. On the conflicting information available, it is difficult to justify the conclusion that stomach or colorectal cancer and asbestos exposure are associated.

## HAEMATOLOGICAL MALIGNANCIES

A link between asbestos exposure and lymphoma and leukaemia has been suggested by Kagan and Jacobson[27] who reported 13 lymphoplasmacytic neoplasms in 13 asbestos workers and reviewed earlier case reports. They speculated that these neoplasms might develop because of alterations of immunological function, such as deficient suppressor T-cell function, in asbestos-exposed people. This type of study is severely limited because of selection bias and a lack of a control group. As about 15% of people in industrialised countries have some exposure to asbestos these findings may be coincidental. No excess of lymphatic and haematological malignancies was found in the UK Health and Safety Executive's mortality survey of British asbestos workers.[2] A recent review by Becker et al.[28] of six cohort and 16 case control studies found that a causal relationship between asbestos exposure and the subsequent development of lymphoma could not be derived from the published results but recommended that future studies should examine more closely the type and severity of asbestos exposures and subclassify the haematological malignancies into the sub-entities.

## CONCLUSIONS

The published data do not justify drawing links between asbestos exposure and laryngeal, gastrointestinal and haematological neoplasms.

### References

1. Tossavainen A. Asbestos, asbestosis and cancer. Exposure criteria for clinical diagnosis. Proceedings of the International Expert Group on Asbestos, Asbestosis and Cancer. *People and Work Research Reports* 1997; **14**: 8–27.
2. Hutchings S, Jones J, Hodgson J. *Asbestos Related Diseases. Decennial Supplement*. London: HMSO, 1996; 127–152.
3. Hodgson J, Darnton A. The quantitative risks of mesothelioma and lung cancer in relation to asbestos exposure. *Ann Occup Hyg* 2000; **44**: 565–601.
4. Lanphear BP, Buncher CR. Latent period for malignant mesothelioma of occupational origin. *J Med* 1992; **34**: 718–721.
5. Carbone M. SV40: from monkeys to humans. *Semin Cancer Biol* 2001; **11**: 1–84.
6. Jasani B, Jones C, Radu C et al. Simian virus 40 detection in human mesothelioma: reliability and significance of the available molecular evidence. *Front Biosci* 1999; **6**: 12–22.
7. Attanoos RL, Gibbs AR. Closed percutaneous and open pleural biopsy diagnosis of malignant pleural mesothelioma (DPM) – an audit from a Regional Thoracic Centre. *Mod Pathol* 2002; **15**: 314A.
8. Gibbs AR, Attanoos RL. Examination of lung specimens. *J Clin Pathol* 2000; **53**: 507–512.
9. Gibbs AR, Pooley FD. Analysis and interpretation of inorganic mineral particles in 'lung tissues'. *Thorax* 1996; **51**: 327–334.
10. Doll R. Mortality from lung cancer in asbestos workers. *Br J Ind Med* 1955; **12**: 81–86.
11. Churg A. Neoplastic asbestos-induced disease. In: Churg A, Green FHY. (eds) *Pathology of Occupational Lung Disease*, 2nd edn. Baltimore, MD: Williams and Wilkins, 1998; 339–392.
12. Steenland K, Loomis D, Shy S et al. Review of occupational lung carcinogens. *Am J Ind Med* 1996; **29**: 474–490.
13. Liddell FKD. The interaction of asbestos and smoking and lung cancer. *Ann Occup Hyg* 2001; **45**: 341–356.
14. Mossman BT, Kamp DW, Weitzman SA. Mechanisms of carcinogenesis and clinical feature of asbestos-associated cancers. *Cancer Invest* 1996; **14**: 466–480.
15. Bohlig J, Jacob G, Muller H. *Die Asbestose der Lunger*. Stuttgart: Georg Thieme, 1960.
16. Sluis-Kremer G, Bezuidenhout BN. Relation between asbestosis and bronchial cancer in amphibole asbestos miners. *Br J Ind Med* 1989; **46**: 537–540.
17. Weiss W. Asbestos and colorectal cancer. *Gastroenterology* 1990; **99**: 876–884.
18. Hughes JM, Weill H. Asbestosis as a precursor of asbestos related lung cancer: results of a prospective mortality study. *Br J Ind Med* 1991; **48**: 229–233.
19. Anon. Consensus report. Asbestos, asbestosis and cancer: the Helsinki criteria and proposed grading schema. *Scand J Work Environ Health* 1997; **23**: 311–316.

20. De Vos Irvine H, Lamont DW, Hole DJ *et al*. Asbestos and lung cancer in Glasgow and the west of Scotland. *BMJ* 1993; **306**: 1503–1506.
21. Karjalainen A, Anttila S, Van Hala E *et al*. Asbestos exposure and the risk of lung cancer in the general urban population. *Scand J Work Environ Health* 1994; **20**: 243–250.
22. Wilkinson P, Hansell DM, Janssens J *et al*. Is lung cancer associated with asbestos exposure when there are no small opacities on the chest radiograph? *Lancet* 1995; **345**: 1074–1078.
23. Wagner JC, Moncrieff CB, Coles R *et al*. Correlation between fibre content of the lungs and disease in naval dockyard workers. *Br J Ind Med* 1986; **43**: 391–395.
24. Muscat JE, Wynder EL. Tobacco, alcohol, asbestos and occupational risk factors for laryngeal cancer. *Cancer* 1992; **69**: 2244–2251.
25. Browne K, Gee JBL. Asbestos exposure and laryngeal cancer. *Ann Occup Hyg* 2000; **44**: 239–250.
26. Kang S, Burnett CA, Freund E *et al*. Gastrointestinal mortality of workers in occupations with high asbestos exposures. *Am J Ind Med* 1997; **31**: 713–718.
27. Kagan E, Jacobson RJ. Lymphoid and plasma cell malignancies – asbestos related disorders of long latency. *Am J Clin Pathol* 1980; **80**: 14–20.
28. Becker N, Berger U, Bolm-Audorff U. Asbestos exposure and malignant lymphomas – a recent review of the epidemiological literature. *Int Arch Occup Environ Health* 2001; **74**: 459–469.

*Franklin V. Peale Jr  Kenneth J. Hillan*

**6**

# Tissue arrays: construction and applications

Less than 5 years ago, Olli Kallioniemi, Guido Sauter and colleagues published their seminal paper describing high-density tissue microarrays (TMAs), a surprisingly robust method for creating a single paraffin block containing hundreds of well-ordered tissue samples, each roughly the diameter of a propelling pencil lead.[1] Since then, TMAs have become a staple of pathology research. Initial scepticism about the capacity of tiny tissue samples to accurately represent the biology of larger disease processes has been resolved. The method has proven particularly powerful for correlating gene and protein expression patterns in intact tissues with clinical outcomes in large patient populations though more prosaic applications, including interlaboratory quality assurance and intralaboratory control standards, will probably make TMAs common in research and routine anatomical pathology practice. The technical barriers to TMA use are low enough that all practising pathologists should consider the technique within their scope.

## TMA CONSTRUCTION

### PRECEDENT

As noted by Kononen *et al.*,[1] the concept of assembling multiple tissues into one well-ordered block predates TMAs. Hector Battifora described 'checkerboard' blocks containing grids of millimetre-square tissue strips embedded in agar and paraffin. He recommended the use of such blocks for quality control and reagent testing, but advised that they were 'not a substitute for conventional

**Dr Franklin V. Peale Jr** MD PhD
Associate Director, Department of Pathology, Genentech, Inc., 1 DNA Way South San Francisco, CA 94080, USA

**Dr Kenneth J. Hillan** MBChB FRCS FRCPath
Vice President, Department of Pathology, Genentech, Inc., MS#72B, 1 DNA Way, South San Francisco, CA 94080, USA (for correspondence)

studies based on larger samples of tissue'.[2] Tissue microarrays refine the checkerboard block concept by assembling needle biopsy cores taken from many paraffin-embedded tissues into one block, reducing the size of the sampled tissue, simplifying the mechanics of block construction, and allowing the donor blocks to be preserved more or less intact. Remarkably, clinical correlations relating tumour stage and patient outcomes with pathological criteria measured in typical 'large section' paraffin specimens can be faithfully reproduced with only 1–4 TMA cores taken from diagnostic tissue. The elegance of the TMA concept belies two general challenges to a TMA user: (i) a mechanical challenge in building an array and cutting satisfactory histological sections from the assembled TMA block; and (ii) an information management challenge in tracking the data associated with each core. Neither is insurmountable but, perhaps surprisingly, the mechanical challenge may be simpler than the data management one.

## ARRAYER MECHANICS

The tissue microarray concept can be implemented with cores of any diameter. Kononen *et al.* chose 0.6 mm as a compromise which permits large numbers of samples to be arranged in a single paraffin wax cassette while still allowing adequate tissue sampling in each core. Assembling the many 0.6 mm paraffin tissue cores at a 0.8–1 mm intercore spacing in a regular grid requires precise control; the tissue cores and the recipient paraffin wax wells are fragile and manual cutting and placing of cores is impractical. Adequate results can be had (if slowly) with a 3-axis stereotactic needle holder and a punch biopsy set, but commercially available tissue arrayers are routinely used.

The first available and still most widely used arrayer, built by Beecher Instruments (see Table 1 for sources of TMA-related hardware and software), permits micrometre-controlled X–Y axis block positioning with manual vertical punch/stylet control. The Beecher tissue arrayer uses two core punches with different diameters: the smaller punch is used to make wells in the recipient block. It has an outside diameter approximately equal to the inside diameter of the second larger punch, which is used to cut tissue cores from the donor block.[3] Chemicon and Alphelys also recently offered manual arrayers of slightly different designs, and a second-generation automated arrayer is available from Beecher Instruments. Remarkably, the process of punching tissue cores from a donor block produces no significant distortion either in the tissue core or in the donor block. Multiple cores can be removed from donor blocks without compromising the remaining tissue. Because TMA cores can be taken in replicates from the donor block, multiple arrays can be built even from relatively rare clinical material. This ability effectively to 'clone' the donor paraffin wax block allows correspondingly increased numbers of parallel assays to be done on a single tissue sample.

Frozen tissue arrays have also been described[4] though the mechanics of making and using these is more challenging. Fejzo and Slamon assembled their frozen arrays using the Beecher arrayer by cooling the working parts with dry ice. These authors note that sampling tissue frozen in OCT must be done slowly to avoid breaking punches (1.0 mm diameter punches are sturdier than 0.6 mm punches) and that Instrumedic's slide adhesive system (see Table 1) is

**Table 1** TMA hardware and software resources

| | |
|---|---|
| **TMA imaging hardware** | |
| Universal Imaging Corp. | www.image1.com/products/tma/ |
| ChromaVision Medical Systems | |
| | www.chromavision.com/prod/microtissue/index.htm |
| Bacus Laboratories, Inc. | www.bacuslabs.com/indexbliss.html |
| Aperio Technologies | www.aperio.com/ |
| Alphelys | www.alphelys.com/us/pTA_StationAnalyse.htm |
| | |
| **TMA imaging software** | |
| Commercial | |
| TissueImformatics.Inc | www.bacuslabs.com/bliss.html |
| Aperio Technologies | www.aperio.com/ |
| BioGenex | www.biogenex.com |
| Alphelys | www.alphelys.com/us/pTA_StationAnalyse.htm |
| Academic | |
| van der Rijn laboratory | http://genome-www.stanford.edu/TMA/ |
| | |
| **TMA construction hardware** | |
| Beecher Instruments | www.beecherinstruments.com/ |
| Chemicon International, Inc. | |
| | www.chemicon.com/Featured/ata100-Arrayer.asp |
| | |
| **TMA slides** | |
| Commercial | |
| ZyMed Laboratories Inc. | www.zymed.com/ |
| BioGenex | www.biogenex.com |
| Clinomics Biosciences Inc. | |
| | www.clinomicslabs.net/catalogs/tissue_micro_array.asp |
| Ambion, Inc | www.ambion.com/catalog/ |
| Academic | |
| National Cancer Institute Tissue Array | |
| Research Program (TARP) | http://resresources.nci.nih.gov/tarp/ |
| | www-cbctr.ims.nci.nih.gov/applic.html |
| Cooperative Human Tissue | |
| Network (CHTN) | http://faculty.virginia.edu/chtn-tma/index.html |
| | |
| **TMA data exchange standards (proposed)** | |
| Jules J. Berman, Mary E. Edgerton, | |
| Bruce A. Friedman *et al*. | www.pathinfo.com/jjb/tmafaqv1.htm |
| | |
| **TMA data handling** | |
| van der Rijn laboratory | http://genome-www.stanford.edu/TMA/ |
| Cattoretti laboratory | http://ICG.cpmc.columbia.edu/cattoretti/Protocol/ |
| | Immunohistochemistry/TissueArray.html |
| Genentech Pathology | www.interscience.wiley.com/jpages/ |
| | 0022-3417/license.html |

essential to hold the cores in place when sectioning. In our own laboratory, we found the frozen OCT matrix too hard for routine use of the Beecher arrayer, but we have been successful with manual cutting, using 1 mm bore needles and larger inter-core spacing. In our experience, the Instrumedic tape system resulted in extensive freeze-thaw artefact whereas sections cut without the tape system had very good morphology. Bonding of cores to the surrounding OCT block was facilitated by keeping in a cryostat slightly warmer than usual at −16°C. Figure 1 illustrates a frozen array built in this way. Immuno-histochemistry, mRNA ISH and chromosomal FISH can be performed successfully using frozen tissue arrays.[4]

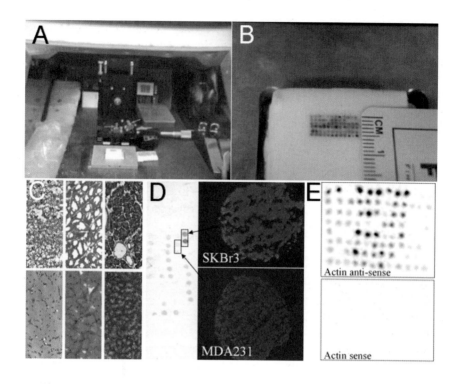

**Fig. 1** (A) A Beecher tissue arrayer, designed for room temperature use with paraffin-embedded tissues, can be adapted to cut frozen tissue cores, either by cooling the necessary components with dry ice (see Fejzo & Slamon[4]) or by installing the arrayer in a cryotome, as illustrated here. Frozen tissue, being much harder than paraffin, requires slow cutting with increased mechanical force. (B) Detail of an assembled frozen tissue array constructed of 0.6 mm cores at 1 mm core spacing. (C) Histological sections cut from a frozen array using either the Instrumedic tape system (upper 3 panels) or without the tape system (lower 3 panels). In our experience, better results are obtained by cutting frozen TMAs directly onto glass slides. With practice, core retention, even without the use of adhesive tape, can approach 80%. (D) Detail of a phosphorimager low magnification scan (black and white image, left panel) and high magnification fluorescence image from the same array after immunostaining with anti-Her2. SKBr3 breast cancer cells expressing approximately $2.4 \times 10^6$ Her2 molecules/cell are brightly stained, whereas MDA231 cells expressing only $2.2 \times 10^4$ Her2 molecules/cell appear unstained. (E) Detail of a phosphorimager scan of an isotopic *in situ* hybridization result. Glass slides hybridized with $[^{33}P]$-labelled riboprobes are exposed to low-energy storage phosphor screens, which are then imaged. As expected, signal intensity varies across tissue cores hybridized with antisense (AS) riboprobes; tissue cores hybridized with control sense (S) riboprobes show no signal. The location of tissue cores that hybridize weakly or not at all can be determined by scanning the same glass slides directly in fluorescence mode; tissue autofluorescence is a reliable indicator of core location and integrity.

## TISSUE SELECTION

Whatever mechanism is used to build the array, someone must first identify and collect the appropriate donor paraffin wax blocks, examine representative H&E-stained sections of the donor tissue, mark on an H&E slide the area of interest to be included in the TMA, and transfer the marked slide and paraffin wax block to the person who will build the array. There are few limitations to tissue selection though ideally donor blocks should contain a 2–3 mm thickness of the target tissue to permit the greatest number of serial histological section to be cut from the TMA block. Control of core placement depth in the recipient block is important; ideally, all cores should contain tissue of the same depth and should be positioned so that the tissues begin and end in two planes parallel to the block face. Without this condition, TMA sections cut from the beginning and end of a block will contain variable numbers of 'empty' core positions reflecting the variable core lengths. Tissue arrayer punches can be fitted with depth stops to help the user control the vertical core placement. A single, well-made TMA can routinely yield 100–300 sections before the number of exhausted cores makes the array unusable.

## TMA CORE SIZE

Not surprisingly, tissue heterogeneity and the small size of the arrayed cores (the diameter of a 0.6 mm core just fills the field of view of a typical 40x objective) are immediate concerns for most pathologists first considering the technique. A typical 'large section' histology cassette may represents only 0.05% of the total tumour volume (assuming 1 cassette per cubic centimetre of tumour), and a typical TMA core represents just 0.3% of this amount.[5] It is not intuitively obvious that the sample of tissue present in a TMA core is adequate for diagnostic purposes. This premise has, however, been rigorously proven for many applications.[1,5–7] The diagnostic utility of any TMA core depends on sampling representative donor tissue sites and having sample replicates adequate for the diagnostic question at hand. For practical purposes, some tissues are easier to sample than others: relatively uniform solid tissues present fewer challenges than tissues with large-scale architectural variations (*e.g.* lymph nodes, GI tract) or tissues with microscopically fine diagnostic features (*e.g.* epithelial, mucosal and serosal surfaces). Careful marking and orientation of the donor blocks and increased sampling can allow TMAs yielding 100 or more representative sections even from tissues with complex architecture.[1]

## ARRAY DESIGN

When scoring TMAs microscopically, it is easy to lose one's place when there are more than 10 cores in either axis. Some users (*e.g.* the National Cancer Institute TARP) group cores in large arrays into sub-arrays of smaller dimensions (*e.g.* 5 rows, 5 columns) with 'empty' spaces between successive sub-arrays. Marker cores of various types can be placed to help to orientate the array unambiguously, keep track of one's place when reading slides, or to control for satisfactory experimental technique. Many users include marker cores cut from a characteristic tissue type,[8] coloured crayon, or other material. We have used a 50/50 (v/v) mixture of 2% low melting temperature agarose and surgical marking ink, processed routinely and embedded in paraffin wax. Asymmetric placement of marker cores assures unambiguous orientation of the arrays.

Cores designed as positive and negative controls for specific assays can also be incorporated into arrays. These could include samples of tissue culture cell lines expressing known levels of specific genes,[9] generic cell lines transfected with specific cDNAs in appropriate expression vectors, agarose cores containing known amounts of specific, *in vitro* transcribed RNA, DNA or purified protein, or material that non-specifically binds isotopic nucleic acids (*e.g.* cellulose fibres). The latter cores can be used to help align autoradiographic film or phosphorimager images of isotopic ISH results with core maps.

Some thought should be given to the placement of cores in the array, depending on the study design. Replicate cores from the same donor block can be grouped together for ease of interpretation; other users prefer to distribute them across the entire array or to independent replicate arrays. Distribution of similar samples controls for regional variation in staining or hybridization efficiency and makes scoring of replicate cores more independent. Different disease processes included in a single block can similarly be grouped or dispersed: clustering similar specimens in one area of the array facilitates rapid overall interpretation of staining results but offers the possibility that regional variations in detection efficiency will affect one disease type more than another. A hybrid solution is to cluster replicate cores and disease processes, but to include internal control cores to assess technical adequacy in different regions of the block.

## SECTIONING ARRAYS

TMA cores are slip-fit into recipient block holes, without any added bonding material between the cores and the surrounding paraffin wax. Consequently, sections cut from the block face have little to hold the cores in place. Many users rely on sectioning aids such as the Instrumedics tape/adhesive slide system (Table 1). One disadvantage of this system is that the adhesive material between the glass slide and histological section causes some optical distortion; this is generally not a significant problem for routine bright-field interpretation, but dark field images are adversely affected. Alternatively, the completed TMA block can be 'annealed', covered by a metal embedding mould, in an oven at 37°C for 24 h, then 50°C for 10 min. This step softens the paraffin wax in the cores and surrounding block enough to permit bonding. Sections cut from annealed blocks retain cores effectively without the assistance of tape sectioning aids. If TMAs are assembled from donor blocks obtained from multiple institutions, or from one institution over many years, cores with more than one formulation of paraffin wax may be brought into a single TMA. Ideally, the melting temperature and hardness of the donor and recipient block blocks' paraffin wax should match. Despite their small size, TMA cores adhere fastidiously to microscope slides (we routinely use Fisher brand 'Plus' slides) without requiring special pretreatments even in the course of more aggressive handling (protease digestion, high temperatures, formamide solvent) necessary for *in situ* hybridization, immunohistochemistry and FISH analysis. In one published TMA FISH study, 75–85% of cores yielded interpretable results; only two-thirds of the uninterpretable results were due to problems related to the TMA technique, most commonly absence of core tissue in the section, and lack of adequate tumour in the core tissue; TMA cores fell off the slide during processing only 2% of the time.[10]

Assembling a TMA requires patience and skill well within the abilities of a good histotechnologist and is not a trivial effort. In respect of the effort, all possible sections that can be cut from the block should be obtained, stored and used as conservatively as possible. Section yield is maximized by cutting the entire TMA block in one sitting, storing all slides obtained for future use. An important caveat applies: while antigenicity of tissue stored in paraffin wax blocks can be retained for up to 70 years,[5] some epitopes degrade on storage of unstained histological sections. Decreased staining intensity or percent tissue reactivity or both has been documented for p53, oestrogen receptor, androgen receptor, Factor VIII, bcl-2, chromogranin, CD3, Ki67, EGFR and PSA immunoreactivity.[11–14] We have found significant degradation of VEGF reactivity to R&D Systems clone 293 antibody over relatively short intervals of storage at room temperature in room air. Some changes are reportedly slowed by storage at reduced temperature[12] or increased primary antibody concentrations.[14] On the reasonable assumption that antigen oxidation is, at least in part, responsible, some laboratories store cut TMA sections under nitrogen or after re-coating the glass-mounted section in paraffin wax,[5] though the latter precaution has been shown to be ineffective in some cases.[12] For applications other than immunohistochemistry, the risk of signal loss during routine storage are less well documented. We have used tissue sections stored more than 1 year under ambient conditions for mRNA *in situ* hybridization analysis without noticeable loss of signal.

## EVALUATING MOLECULAR MARKERS IN TMAS

TMAs were originally designed for large-scale molecular marker studies in paraffin wax embedded tissues using semi-quantitative scoring systems. The reproducibility of this, and other analytical approaches, is facilitated by including cell line or synthetic controls in the original TMA design, or by preparing small cell pellet arrays that can be placed on the slide alongside the original TMA section. Incorporation of standard controls also allows comparison of experiments carried out at different times and in different laboratories. Combining speech recognition software with a text-to-speech soundproofing tool can facilitate recording results from a large series of arrays. This enables a pathologist to enter data directly into a spreadsheet or database without having to look up from the microscope. Reliable entry of data at a rate of 1 tissue element per second can be achieved by this means.

For image capture, we use a semi-automated system, based on a Nikon Eclipse E1000 microscope, that can image 8 slides on a single run in each of bright-field, dark-field and three colour fluorescent modes. The system transfers the captured images to a relational database for on-line review by pathologists and their collaborators. Images can also be subjected to batch-mode morphometric analysis using software packages such as MetaMorph® or NIH Image.

For isotopic, *in situ* hybridization analysis, we use a phosphorimager for high throughput quantitative analysis (Fig. 2). This method correlates well with other quantitative techniques (*e.g.* Taqman) and can be completed within 24 h of hybridization, as opposed to the usual 2–4 weeks. Measurement is objective and has greater dynamic range than traditional semi-quantitative evaluation by eye. Similar quantitative technologies have been applied for immunofluorescence detection of proteins and or nucleic acids.[15]

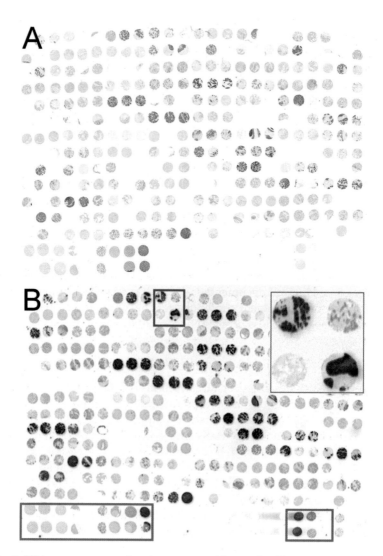

**Fig. 2** (A) Low power scan of an immunoperoxidase stained breast cancer TMA using an anti-HER2 antibody that recognises the extracellular domain (ECD) of HER2. The bottom two rows include, on the left, duplicate cell pellet controls and, on the right, synthetic agarose controls containing decreasing concentrations of HER2 ECD.
(B) A section from the same array, stained with the same anti-HER2 primary antibody, using an Alexa Fluor® 647 labelled conjugate for secondary detection. The section was scanned using a cDNA microarray scanner with 3 μm resolution. The blue-boxed inset demonstrates the resolution that can be attained. Red boxes outline the cell pellets (left) and agarose-protein ECD controls (right) can be used to generate protein standard concentration curves. Fluorescent detection combines the advantages of increase detection sensitivity with a more truly quantitative a signal that is linear over a 5-log range.

## TMA INFORMATICS – SOURCE TISSUE DATA MANAGEMENT

The TMA technique implies an ordered arrangement of cores in the recipient block; it imposes on the user a data management challenge that is arguably more daunting than the mechanics of building and sectioning the array. A large tissue array can contain up to 1000 cores, each of which has invariant source data that must be recorded – minimally, core tissue and pathological diagnosis. Additional information can be patient-specific (demographics, disease stage, treatment history), tissue-specific (tissue type and pathological diagnosis), and core-specific (including location within the donor tissue – tumour centre, tumour margin, normal tissue adjacent to tumour). The core tissue and pathological diagnosis may be different from the tissue and diagnosis of the larger donor block (*e.g.* when sampling normal tissue adjacent to tumour) or tissue subsets in a heterogeneous organ (*e.g.* lymphoid tissue in bowel). Metastatic disease is a special case; data for both the tissue of disease origin and tissue in which the metastasis resides should be clearly recorded.

## TMA INFORMATICS – RESULTS DATA MANAGEMENT

In addition to source tissue information, each TMA block can be used to generate hundreds of experimental slides, each core of which will have one or more result data points. For example, a single IHC experiment could generate four data types: (i) quantitative (a fluorescence intensity or phosphorimager value); (ii) discrete semiquantitative (a pathologist's score); (iii) free text (a comment on the result); or (iv) image (data that could include one or more magnifications and illumination modes –fluorescent, bright-field, dark-field). A modestly sized (200-core) TMA block yielding 100 useful sections would generate 20,000 data points even if only one result were recorded for each core in each section. Ideally, the software design should allow all data related to cores taken from a single donor tissue block, even if used in multiple different TMA designs, to be retrieved for comparison.

Many TMA laboratories have developed data management tools of increasing sophistication using personal computer-based spreadsheet or database software (*e.g.* Microsoft Excel or Access). These programs are particularly well-suited for 'smaller' data sets (Excel allows 65,535 rows and 255 columns in one spreadsheet). Comprehensive applications integrating image acquisition, data acquisition and statistical analysis have been built around these frameworks.[8,16] Relational databases capable of handling larger data sets have been built at other institutions. Most solutions include graphical representations ('maps') of core locations in the array, both for assistance in designing the array and in reading results from slides. Many systems store individual core images (usually compressed) for later review, often via a web browser.[16,17] To assure unbiased interpretation of results, some groups prefer to do TMA scoring 'anonymously' (*i.e.* with minimal experimental and core data available) via such web interfaces. Review of stored images also allows scoring disparities between users to be mediated rapidly. Image storage and retrieval increases the data storage and handling demands of a TMA information management system exponentially. Several excellent software packages are in the public domain, and others are commercially available (see Table 1).

## TMA INFORMATICS – DATA EXCHANGE

There has been some discussion, but as yet no universal consensus, on the appropriate way to exchange TMA data. One immediate need is for academic and commercial suppliers of TMA slides to provide source-tissue information to the end-user. Most TMA source laboratories provide 'maps' with corresponding tissue/diagnosis data, but the data formats and media vary widely (paper copies, HTML pages, Excel spreadsheets). A commonly accepted minimal standard for sharing TMA core source information would facilitate the wider use of arrays produced in different institution. Sharing of result data is a more challenging problem. To interpret and use data generated in another institution properly, details of experimental conditions, assay instrumentation, scoring criteria, and other experimental variables should be provided along with the data sets themselves. The data sets can be shared easily only if the institutions use the same software or if they have a common data exchange standard. Discussions among interested TMA investigators in the US has resulted in the creation of a preliminary XML data exchange working standard.[18]

## TMA APPLICATIONS

The high density of tissue samples on a single TMA slide permits high volume, well-controlled parallel histological assays to be performed with a minimum of reagent and effort. The entire range of routine tissue-based analyses, including immunohistochemistry, mRNA *in situ* hybridization (ISH) and chromosomal fluorescence *in situ* hybridization (FISH), have been done successfully on TMAs. The original authors[1] emphasize that despite the small size of the sampled tissue in TMA cores, with adequate core replicates (often less than 4), TMA data usually confirm clinical-pathological correlations obtained with larger tissue analyses. The increased statistical power inherent in the large tissue sample numbers has revealed new clinical pathological correlations.

### CORRELATION OF TMA DATA WITH 'LARGE SECTION' DATA

Several early TMA studies rigorously addressed the concern that the small size of TMA cores would not allow representative evaluation of the larger tissue biology. Kononen *et al.* presented data in the first TMA paper that core-based IHC correlated with tissue homogenate ER measurements in 84% of TMA cores, comparable to the correlation obtained between tissue homogenates and large section IHC.[1] Rimm and colleagues measured ER, PR and Her2 protein by IHC in 36 cases of breast cancer in TMAs and large sections from the same cases.[5] In > 97% of cases, breast cancer TMA samples were concordant with the whole-section IHC analysis. For all three diagnostic proteins, two TMA cores per tissue sample gave a > 95% likelihood, and four cores gave a > 98% likelihood that the TMA cores would accurately reflect the immunostaining pattern of the entire tissue sample.[5] A similar analysis compared histological grading of bladder tumours, which may be even more subjective than IHC positivity, in TMA cores and large sections.[7] Bladder tumour grade measured in large tissue sections was accurately reflected by the maximum tumour grade observed in four TMA cores. TMA core maximum tumour grade correlated as well as large section tumour grade with patient disease-specific survival and progression-free survival.[7]

## CORRELATION OF PROTEIN EXPRESSION WITH CLINICAL OUTCOME

When protein expression data from TMA tissue samples are linked to disease stage and particularly to clinical outcomes data, they allow powerful epidemiological analyses. Immunohistochemical staining of ER, PR and p53 expression in 553 breast cancer specimens from patients with clinical follow-up allowed Torhorst *et al.* to compare 'large section' and TMA-based expression data relative to patient survival.[6] Remarkably, ER expression across this population, even when measured in a single TMA core, accurately reflected the ER expression of the population measured in large histological sections. More importantly, clinical survival correlated equally with measured ER levels, whether one TMA core or four TMA cores were evaluated per patient, and both were equivalent to large section analysis.[6] Similar data were obtained for PR and p53 expression, though for these proteins measurements on four cores more accurately reflected the results obtained for large section analysis. Remarkably, p53 expression as measured in TMA cores was better correlated with survival than the same analysis done in large tissue sections. The authors argue that TMA cores may provide a more reliable estimate of the overall pattern of gene expression in the tumour; by presenting a limited 'target' for the pathologist to interpret, the TMA cores prevent the pathologist from subjectively interpreting a large sample with one pattern according to an alternate staining pattern present only in a subset of tumour cells.[6] In a more recent study, telomerase hTERT and hTR subunit expression were measured in 611 breast cancer samples; high expression of either component was associated with decreased survival and hTERT expression was an independent prognostic factor.[19] Where possible, we include the construction of tissue arrays from tumour blocks of patients enrolled in clinical trials to assess which molecular markers might predict response or resistance to targeted therapies.

## FISH ANALYSIS OF GENE AMPLIFICATION

FISH analysis on TMA tissue was first demonstrated in the original paper by Kononen *et al.*, in which 372 primary breast cancer samples were analyzed for *HER2*, *MYC*, and *CCCND1* gene amplification; results on TMA samples were consistent with published values obtained with larger tissue sections.[1] Tumours with *HER2* gene amplification were found by parallel IHC analysis to have Her2 protein overexpression, as expected.[1] The same group explored the correlation between disease progression and gene amplification in prostate cancer.[20] In a survey of 371 prostate samples, androgen receptor amplification was found in 22–23% of hormone refractory tumours, whether locally recurrent or metastatic, significantly more common than the 1% and 0% amplification rate seen in primary tumours and nodular prostatic hypertrophy, respectively. *MYC* gene amplification was significantly more common in metastatic disease (11%) than in locally recurrent disease (4%). On the other hand, the authors were not able to support a previously reported amplification of *HER2* in prostate cancer.[20] In a survey of gene amplification in many tumour types, the same authors measured *HER2*, *MYC* and *CCCND1* gene amplification in 397 tumour samples representing 17 disease processes.[10] Tumour-specific gene amplifications previously described in the literature were confirmed in 16 of 25 diseases (64%) in which fewer than 25 cases were examined, but in 11 of 12 diseases (92%) in which more than 25 tissue samples were examined.[10] The same group examined 372 breast cancers for amplification of 6 specific genes clustered near 17q2321 and 4788 tissues representing 206 different disease process for amplification of the 17q23 locus near the *TBX* gene.[22] Together, these studies confirmed the utility of TMAs for the rapid evaluation of multigene amplification in large numbers of tissue sample. Because of the technique's high throughput, the latter study showed frequent 17q23 amplification with several tumours (thyroid carcinoma, dermatofibrosarcoma, adenocarcinoma of the ampulla of Vater) not previously recognized to be associated with gene amplification at this locus, and showed statistically significant increased 17q23 amplification in metastatic *versus* primary tumours in adenocarcinoma of the colon, ductal carcinoma of breast and prostate.[22]

## DNA MICROARRAY/TISSUE MICROARRAY SYNERGY

Several groups have productively combined cDNA or oligonucleotide microarray gene expression analysis with tissue microarray analysis. In this strategy, expression profiles for thousands of genes are measured with DNA arrays in a relatively limited number of normal and diseased tissue samples. Candidate genes whose expression appears to differ in these samples are then examined in hundreds of tissues in TMAs, typically by immuno-histochemistry. In the first report of this kind, Bubendorf and co-workers[23] surveyed 5184 genes for those expressed more highly in a hormone-refractory prostate cancer cell line than in its hormone-sensitive parental cell line. Among the most highly up-regulated genes was insulin-like growth factor binding protein 2 (IGFBP2). In the subsequent TMA analysis of 264 clinical prostate tissue samples, IGFBP2 protein was found to be highly expressed in 100% of 30 locally recurrent hormone-refractory tumours, but only in 36% of the 204 primary tumours, and in none of 26 non-neoplastic prostate specimens.[23] This group took a similar approach with renal cell carcinoma (RCC), identifying vimentin up-regulation in the renal carcinoma cell line CRL-1933 relative to normal kidney tissue. Follow-up TMA analysis in 483 renal tumours confirmed overexpression of vimentin in 51–61% of clear cell and papillary RCC, but uncommonly in oncocytoma or chromophobe RCC. These results were consistent with previously reported data from traditional 'large section' studies in smaller patient series. Furthermore, vimentin expression in RCC was found to be a predictor of poor survival in clear cell RCC (383 patients), independent of stage and grade,[24] a result not previously recognized from smaller studies in RCC.

Using a similar strategy, Rubin, Chinnaiyan and colleagues noted increased expression of the enhancer of zeste homologue 2 (EZH2) gene, encoding a transcription factor of the polycomb family, in metastatic *versus* localized prostate cancer. Follow-up analysis of protein expression changes in prostate tissue TMAs revealed increased expression in metastatic disease *versus* benign prostate or localized prostate cancer.[25] Increased EZH2 protein expression in local disease was significantly associated with increased risk of disease recurrence.

## Points for best practice

- The TMA method has become integral to pathology research, if not practice.

- TMA tissue sampling, though limited, is adequate to allow significant clinical correlations.

- Technical hurdles to building and using arrays are not high. Histological quality is not compromised in paraffin wax. Routine staining, IHC, mRNA ISH, DNA FISH techniques do not need modification.

- TMA scoring benefits include: (i) consistent staining/assay on all cores; (ii) rapid evaluation on discrete areas with better uniformity of interpretation; and (iii) reduced subjectivity of selecting tissue area.

- The information management hurdle for using TMAs, beyond the simpler applications, can be significant, but public domain data management tools are available from several sources.

## ACKNOWLEDGEMENTS

We thank Dr A.M. Hanby, Department of Pathology, University of Leeds, UK, for his collaboration on the expression of *HER2* in breast cancer, Stacy Rummonds and Belinda Cairns for their work on frozen TMA techniques.

## References

1. Kononen J, Bubendorf L, Kallioniemi A *et al.* Tissue microarrays for high-throughput molecular profiling of tumour specimens. *Nat Med* 1998; **4**: 844–847.
2. Battifora H, Mehta P. The checkerboard tissue block. An improved multitissue control block. *Lab Invest* 1990; **63**: 722–724.
3. Anon. Instruction Manual, Beecher Instruments Tissue Arrayer. 1998.
4. Fejzo MS, Slamon DJ. Frozen tumor tissue microarray technology for analysis of tumor RNA, DNA, and proteins. *Am J Pathol* 2001; **159**: 1645–1650.
5. Camp RL, Charette LA, Rimm DL. Validation of tissue microarray technology in breast carcinoma. *Lab Invest* 2000; **80**: 1943–1949.
6. Torhorst J, Bucher C, Kononen J *et al.* Tissue microarrays for rapid linking of molecular changes to clinical endpoints. *Am J Pathol* 2001; **159**: 2249–2256.
7. Nocito A, Bubendorf L, Maria Tinner E *et al.* Microarrays of bladder cancer tissue are highly representative of proliferation index and histological grade. *J Pathol* 2001; **194**: 349–357.
8. Liu CL, Prapong W, Natkunam Y *et al.* Software tools for high-throughput analysis and archiving of immunohistochemistry staining data obtained with tissue microarrays. *Am J Pathol* 2002; **161**: 1557–1565.
9. Riera J, Simpson JF, Tamayo R, Battifora H. Use of cultured cells as a control for quantitative immunocytochemical analysis of estrogen receptor in breast cancer. The Quicgel method. *Am J Clin Pathol* 1999; **111**: 329–335.
10. Schraml P, Kononen J, Bubendorf L *et al.* Tissue microarrays for gene amplification surveys in many different tumor types. *Clin Cancer Res* 1999; **5**: 1966–1975.
11. Prioleau J, Schnitt SJ. p53 antigen loss in stored paraffin slides. *N Engl J Med* 1995; **332**: 1521–1522.

12. Jacobs TW, Prioleau JE, Stillman IE, Schnitt SJ. Loss of tumor marker-immunostaining intensity on stored paraffin slides of breast cancer. *J Natl Cancer Inst* 1996; **88**: 1054–1059.

13. Bertheau P, Cazals-Hatem D, Meignin V *et al*. Variability of immunohistochemical reactivity on stored paraffin slides. *J Clin Pathol* 1998; **51**: 370–374.

14. Olapade-Olaopa EO, Ogunbiyi JO, MacKay EH *et al*. Further characterization of storage-related alterations in immunoreactivity of archival tissue sections and its implications for collaborative multicenter immunohistochemical studies. *Appl Immunohistochem Mol Morphol* 2001; **9**: 261–266.

15. Camp RL, Chung GG, Rimm DL. Automated subcellular localization and quantification of protein expression in tissue microarrays. *Nat Med* 2002; **8**: 1323–1327.

16. Manley S, Mucci NR, De Marzo AM, Rubin MA. Relational database structure to manage high-density tissue microarray data and images for pathology studies focusing on clinical outcome: the prostate specialized program of research excellence model. *Am J Pathol* 2001; **159**: 837–843.

17. Bova GS, Parmigiani G, Epstein JI *et al*. Web-based tissue microarray image data analysis: initial validation testing through prostate cancer Gleason grading. *Hum Pathol* 2001; **32**: 417–427.

18. Berman JJ, Edgerton ME, Friedman BA. The tissue microarray data exchange specification: A community-based, open source tool for sharing tissue microarray data. *BMC Med Inform Decis Mak* 2003; **3**: 5.

19. Poremba C, Heine B, Diallo R *et al*. Telomerase as a prognostic marker in breast cancer: high-throughput tissue microarray analysis of hTERT and hTR. *J Pathol* 2002; **198**: 181–189.

20. Bubendorf L, Kononen J, Koivisto P *et al*. Survey of gene amplifications during prostate cancer progression by high-throughout fluorescence *in situ* hybridization on tissue microarrays. *Cancer Res* 1999; **59**: 803–806.

21. Barlund M, Monni O, Kononen J *et al*. Multiple genes at 17q23 undergo amplification and overexpression in breast cancer. *Cancer Res* 2000; **60**: 5340–5344.

22. Andersen CL, Monni O, Wagner U *et al*. High-throughput copy number analysis of 17q23 in 3520 tissue specimens by fluorescence *in situ* hybridization to tissue microarrays. *Am J Pathol* 2002; **161**: 73–79.

23. Bubendorf L, Kolmer M, Kononen J *et al*. Hormone therapy failure in human prostate cancer: analysis by complementary DNA and tissue microarrays. *J Natl Cancer Inst* 1999; **91**: 1758–1764.

24. Moch H, Schraml P, Bubendorf L *et al*. High-throughput tissue microarray analysis to evaluate genes uncovered by cDNA microarray screening in renal cell carcinoma. *Am J Pathol* 1999; **154**: 981–986.

25. Varambally S, Dhanasekaran SM, Zhou M *et al*. The polycomb group protein EZH2 is involved in progression of prostate cancer. *Nature* 2002; **419**: 624–629.

*Clair du Boulay*

**7**

# Error trapping and error avoidance in histopathology

> *To make no mistakes is not in the power of man; but from their errors and mistakes the wise and good learn wisdom for the future.*

**Plutarch**

In the past few years, histopathologists have been accused of diagnostic or professional incompetence with increasing frequency. There is a growing expectation by the public that there should be a zero error rate in histopathology and cytopathology reporting in both screening and diagnostic services.

## ERROR RATES IN DIAGNOSTIC HISTOPATHOLOGY

There are many areas in histopathology in which the correct diagnosis is not clear-cut, a fact not always appreciated by those outside the speciality. Although surgical pathology is commonly regarded as the gold standard in diagnosis, enabling reliable treatment decisions and benchmarking of clinical diagnoses, this is not necessarily true. The fallibility of diagnostic surgical pathology and the serious harm resulting from mis-diagnosis are well described.[1] A UK questionnaire-based survey of errors in diagnostic histopathology showed that a typical histopathologist probably becomes aware of having made a serious diagnostic error about once a year.[2]

There is an emerging consensus in the literature on background error rates in diagnostic histopathology; the clinically significant error rate is 1–2%.[3–5] Overall, some form of diagnostic error will occur in about 3–4% of cases and an error that is likely to affect patient management in 1.0–1.5% (Table 1). It is also recognised in cytopathology screening that a 'zero error rate' is an unreasonable expectation which cannot be achieved, even with the use of automated re-screening devices.[6]

**Dr Clair du Boulay** MSc(Med Ed) DM FRCPath
Director of Medical Education, Southampton University Hospitals NHS Trust, Tremona Road, Southampton SO16 6YD. E-mail: cedb@soton.ac.uk

**Table 1** Classification of diagnostic errors

| | |
|---|---|
| **Category 1** | A diagnostic error which would have a definite influence on clinical management and possible outcome |
| **Category 2** | A diagnostic misinterpretation or oversight which has the potential to affect clinical management or outcome |
| **Category 3** | A minor discrepancy of disease categorisation likely to be of little clinical significance |

## WHAT SORTS OF ERRORS ARE MADE?

There are two main categories of error: (i) **oversight errors** – where the pathologist has missed significant pathology; and (ii) **misinterpretation errors** – where pathological changes are incorrectly interpreted. Both oversight and misinterpretation errors appear to occur with equal frequency.[3]

In an audit of surgical pathology at Southampton when errors were shown to the original diagnosing pathologist, without exception each pathologist recognised the mistake straight away.[7] This suggests that errors are rarely due to incompetence, lack of knowledge or inability to do the work, and that other factors are likely to be important. One of these might be excessive workload, though there does not appear to be an excess of errors in departments with heavy workloads. However, heavy workload was the most frequently cited cause of error by individuals when asked what they thought caused most errors.[2]

There are several well described areas of high-risk practice, where it is known that pathologists tend to make more mistakes that result in litigation; these are lymphoma, melanoma, prostate needle biopsies and diagnoses given by 'expert' consultants.[8] Locum consultant pathologists make a disproportionately large number of errors in samples from the lymphoreticular system.[1]

Physical impairment of visual function might seem an obvious cause of error and there has been some debate about the role of colour vision in histopathology. Colour-blind people make more mistakes than those with normal colour vision but this can be prevented with the adoption of safe systems of working.[9] There is no evidence that pathologists with inability to distinguish subtle colour hues perform less well than others.[10]

## INDIVIDUAL PROFESSIONAL PERFORMANCE

In order to provide the best quality diagnostic service, all histopathologists should be up-to-date with their specialist knowledge, as well as ensuring they have the right skills and attitudes to manage services, communicate effectively and audit their performance. In the UK, there has been a significant change in the requirements and expectations of the public with regard to the professional performance and accountability of doctors.[11,12] From 2004, the General Medical Council (GMC) will require all doctors in the UK to demonstrate that they are fit to remain on the medical register through the re-validation or re-licensing process. In order to re-validate, doctors will have to adhere to the standards set out in 'Good Medical Practice' and participate successfully in a quality assured

CPD scheme and NHS annual appraisal.[13] These measures will ensure that all pathologists are keeping up-to-date and working accountably. Good pathology practice,[14] elaborated by The Royal College of Pathologists from good medical practice, requires all pathologists to:

- Assure the quality of clinical advice given and associated record keeping
- Ensure the quality and timeliness of pathology reports and clinical advice
- Undertake routine review (audit) of a sample of clinical cases/reports in selected areas
- Show that individual diagnostic patterns compare favourably with their peers
- Offer appropriate treatment, management or diagnostic decision making
- Perform autopsies according to The Royal College of Pathologists' guidelines
- Describe the distribution of their workload and case-mix.

## PROFESSIONAL BEHAVIOUR AND WORKING RELATIONSHIPS

There is good evidence that communication and working relationships are extremely important in ensuring high standards of practice, good patient care and reducing errors.[11,15,16] It is not sufficient to be just diagnostically competent and all pathologists must:

- Be available and willing to communicate and discuss clinical and professional issues with colleagues
- Know their own diagnostic limitations as demonstrated by their referral patterns
- Participate in clinicopathological discussions or multidisciplinary team meetings
- Work well in a team
- Be willing to undertake a peer questionnaire or 360 degree review of practice
- Ensure that there are no tensions relating to private practice, coroner's work or outside commitments.

## IDENTIFYING POOR PERFORMANCE

It is essential to identify under-performing pathologists at an early stage to protect patients and maintain high standards of diagnostic pathology. Error-trapping strategies play a part in this. All pathologists make errors of diagnosis and judgement from time-to-time and this is not necessarily evidence of sub-standard practice. It is important not to confuse uncertainty with incompetence: errors should not be judged in isolation but in the context of the pathologist's overall performance.[1,16] Retrospective slide reviews performed with hindsight knowledge can be biased and these alone should not be used to make judgements about performance. Likewise, poor performance cannot be

**Table 2** Factors that may lead to increased risk of errors and poor performance in histopathology

- Conditions of work, staffing and workload
- Locum working in unfamiliar surroundings[18,19]
- Potential constraints on performance in the laboratory or Trust (*e.g.* facilities, culture)
- Low volume work or case-mix and areas where the pathologist may be working outside his or her expertise[20]
- Isolated or single-handed practice

detected by random case review alone because the background error rate obscures slight differences in individual ability. Performance would have to very poor indeed to be detected by these means.[3] Diagnostic histopathology EQA schemes are primarily educational and are not a reliable way to identify poor performance. The performance of doctors must be assessed using the Cambridge model approach, which applies a range of methods and indicators that take into account both individual competence and the day-to-day work context.[17] Factors that may lead to increased risk of errors and poor performance in histopathology are summarised in Table 2.

## CLINICAL AUDIT

Pathologists are personally responsible for ensuring they practice to the highest standards but they need to work in an organisation with systems that support them in doing this. All pathologists and pathology laboratories should show evidence of reliable and systematised audit practice. On-going review of practice through clinical audit is essential for high standards of patient care and reducing errors. There are several key areas in which audit can be used to monitor diagnostic and service standards and identify and prevent error or patterns of error.[3] Audit can provide information about working practices, consistency of reporting and degree of diagnostic consensus. It can also be used to look at diagnostic accuracy and baseline error rates and provide information about the relation between error and workload or intermittent work patterns with busy and quiet periods. Audit and peer review are useful methods for reducing inaccuracies in reports and can be done either by double reporting all or certain categories of cases, or by using random samples. They are all dependent on robust IT systems where appropriate data can be collected and referred back to pathologists. In the UK at present, most laboratory IT systems are inadequate for diagnostic quality improvement systems.

## SPECIALIST REPORTING

There is evidence that in some areas (*e.g.* paediatric pathology), specialist reporting reduces the number of errors made.[21] There is an increasing clinical demand by specialist centres and cancer services for specialist reporting and this is now the norm in many large teaching hospital departments. It is not always feasible or practical in smaller hospitals where cross-cover cannot be provided by a smaller group of pathologists. Whether specialist or generalist reporting is

**Table 3** Terminology of quality issues

| Quality system | A framework of organisational structure |
|---|---|
| Quality assurance | A management system designed to achieve an acceptable level of service |
| Quality control | The operational techniques and activities used to fulfil the requirements |

done, the principles of clinical audit apply and can help reduce errors.

### Clinical governance and quality improvement systems

*A First Class Service* (1998) set out a framework to achieve high quality patient care and services through the following principles:[22]

- Setting of clear national standards

- Delivery of high quality healthcare through clinical governance underpinned by modernised professional self-regulation and extended life-long learning

- Monitoring of quality standards.

The advent of clinical governance and establishment of the Commission for Health Improvement (CHI) have made an impact in improving quality of patient care and services. Quality improvement systems and systematic audit (Table 3) underpin all pathology services – national laboratory accreditation organisations such as CPA in the UK have been very effective in ensuring that laboratories take a systematic approach to quality both in delivery and management of services.

The permanence of microscope slides and written reports exposes pathologists to an inevitable risk of error detection by review of the material: on the other hand, it also provides material for regular audit and the basis of a quality improvement system. Several models of systematised audit and quality improvement have been described and some of these are summarised in Table 4. They range from a systematic review of a sample of cases to systematic double reporting of all cases.[3,4] Double reporting has been shown to be a cost effective way of error trapping when balanced against litigation costs. There are other benefits including a uniform approach to reporting and consistency in sampling and diagnosis. Similarly, a systematic audit of a random sample of cases showed it to be cost effective and feasible.[23] Such systems of internal quality assurance have important benefits in creating a safety culture in the pathology service. They result in more frequent case consultation, uniformity of reporting, collective decision-making about quality and improved feedback to scientific staff. Routine detection of errors prevents harm to patients.

## CONSISTENCY IN REPORTING

In histopathology, the final report is the professional opinion of an individual based on his or her experience and judgement. It is inevitably subjective.

**Table 4** Examples of internal quality processes in diagnostic histopathology

| Type of review | Process |
| --- | --- |
| Intradepartmental consultation | Review of selected cases by colleagues |
| Intra-operative consultation (frozen section) | Review of frozen section diagnosis in the light of final paraffin wax section diagnosis |
| Random case review | Re-reporting of a random sample from all cases submitted |
| Clinical indicator audit | Cases selected on a clinical basis checked over a given period to ensure consistency in diagnosis and reporting |
| Multidisciplinary team meetings (MDTs) | Review of cases presented at all MDTs; comparison of presented diagnosis against reported diagnosis |
| Inter-institutional review | Comparison of local diagnoses with outside review diagnoses |
| Consistency and standards of reporting | Review of cases against standards in datasets and other reporting templates |
| Reporting patterns | Comparison of patterns of reporting among a group of pathologists (e.g. Dukes' staging for colorectal cancer) |
| Workload profile Turnaround times | Audit of busy and quiet periods, case-mix Audit of time taken to produce reports |
| Specimen adequacy | Monitoring identification and processing of specimens |
| Lost specimens | Monitoring number of lost specimens |
| Histology quality control | Assessment of times of delivery of slides and quality of staining |

Observer-dependent morphological features are difficult to standardise and it is well known that there is both inter- and intra-observer variation in diagnostic pathology. The 'correct' diagnosis is not well defined in areas such as lymphoma, Dukes' staging and CIN grading. The greatest inconsistency among reporting pathologists is not usually in the reliability of recognising the entity, but in quantifying degrees of interpretation (*e.g.* grade of tumour, depth of invasion).[1] Errors can be reduced if standardised protocols for diagnostic criteria and sampling are introduced.

## PATTERNS OF ERROR

Random review, systematic audit and double reporting are the mainstays of histopathology error trapping. Another strategy that can be used is to describe reporting patterns so that rather than looking for errors at the individual case level, or at the level of small numbers of selected cases, the observed rate of a pathologist's diagnoses is compared to a known standard or to those of peers or colleagues.[24] This approach could be used as a screening technique for diagnostic variation in pathology.[8] For example, if comparison of the diagnoses of one pathologist with those of a group of other pathologists is very different, this needs to be looked at and questions answered. Does this mean that the pathologist is using different diagnostic criteria and, if so, can this be addressed? This raises questions about when diagnostic variation becomes error and how much variation is acceptable and how much does it affect patient outcomes. It is clear that when large numbers of pathologists report large numbers of cases, the variation will increase, making it very important to develop standardised diagnostic criteria and benchmarking data. Aberrant reporting patterns do not necessarily mean a pathologist is making errors. The analysis of diagnostic patterns shows that specialists frequently over-report malignancy. Diagnostic pattern analysis highlights differences of interpretation and standards, but not the reasons for them. It is a useful early warning system to reveal individuals who are using inappropriate or inconsistent terminology or issuing erroneous reports.

## CASE REFERRAL

Inter- and intra-departmental referral is a time-honoured, usually informal way in which pathologists ask for another opinion or check out their diagnosis with a colleague or peer. Both have a significant and measurable impact on the quality of diagnostic pathology.[25,26] They are useful ways of preventing error and constitute good practice as well as reflecting a culture in which pathologists can admit to uncertainty and their own limitations and communicate with colleagues.

## MULTIDISCIPLINARY TEAM MEETINGS (MDTS)

The clinicopathological meeting or MDT has for many histopathologists always been an important part of their professional practice. The MDT is now routine and commonplace, and a requirement of being part of a cancer centre or network. The MDT is a forum for case discussion and review of clinical and pathological material. Pathologists, clinicians, nurses, members of the cancer team, technical staff and radiologists may attend. Clinical decisions are made and acted upon, and errors or potential errors dealt with before they can affect the patient. The clinical team provides clinical context and feedback for the pathologist and any outcomes and changed diagnoses are recorded for audit purposes. This is a good way of maintaining the quality of histopathology reports and also provides a proxy marker of patterns of reporting for pathologists. Those with a high rate of changed diagnosis may have cause for concern. The MDT is a cost effective way of error trapping and quality improvement.[27] Sessions for MDTs should be part of every pathologist's job plan and contract of employment. Modification of diagnosis at MDTs occurs at a higher rate than could be detected by routine audit and regular MDTs or diagnostic slide review sessions result in a reduced rate of amended final reports.[28]

## USE OF GUIDELINES AND DATASETS

The use of datasets and national guidelines is a good way to ensure consistency of diagnostic criteria and standards. Increasing numbers of these are nationally available, produced by the Department of Health, National Institute for Clinical Excellence (NICE) and professional bodies such as The Royal College of Pathologists and specialist societies. All pathologists should adhere to and apply national practice guidelines. The Royal College of Pathologists has published a series of minimum datasets for histopathology reporting in cancer and these, along with other reporting templates, have been shown to be very effective.[29]

## EXTERNAL QUALITY ASSURANCE (EQA)

Diagnostic laboratories use EQA schemes to maintain their standards and to benchmark themselves with other centres. EQA schemes are also used in the area of interpretative histopathology. In the UK there are now many local, regional and national schemes available; some of these are general and others specialist. Some are organised as 'slide clubs'; others are more formal, accredited and have scoring systems. Interpretative EQA schemes are educationally valuable and as such are recognised for CPD credits by The Royal College of Pathologists. The process of looking at slides, discussing them with colleagues and then receiving feedback and comparison with peers is important. It must be emphasised that although scores are frequently given, they are not a direct measure of competence or performance. However a pathologist who consistently scores below an agreed standard, or refuses to participate in a scheme, would be a cause for concern.

## RISK MANAGEMENT

Clinical risk management is about identifying what goes wrong in patient care and why, and learning lessons from these events to ensure action is taken to prevent recurrence. Organisations need to create a culture of openness, so that staff are not afraid to report untoward events and lessons may be learnt and implemented.

In 2002, the UK National Patient Safety Agency (NPSA) estimated that 850,000 adverse incidents occur each year in the NHS, translating to an estimate that 1 in 10 patients are subject to some kind of medical 'error' or iatrogenic event. *An Organisation With a Memory*[30] makes it clear that the NHS should develop and foster a culture where it is recognised that clinicians will make mistakes, but where systems are in place to minimise their impact on patients. Successful safety-conscious organisations such as the airline industry recognise that human fallibility is inevitable and so develop systems to avert errors, being constantly pre-occupied with the possibility of failure. There are two approaches to human fallibility – the person and the system approaches. The first focuses on the errors of individuals, blaming them for forgetfulness, inattention or moral weakness; the second concentrates on the conditions under which individuals work and tries to build defences to avert errors or mitigate their effects. The systems approach recognises the factors of the 'vulnerable system syndrome' which comprises three interacting and self-perpetuating elements[31] which is essentially a recipe for disaster:

- Blaming front-line staff
- Denying the existence of systematic and error-provoking weaknesses
- Blinkered pursuit of productive and financial indicators.

## ADVERSE INCIDENT REPORTING

The NPSA is a special health authority created to co-ordinate the efforts of all those involved in healthcare and to learn from adverse incidents occurring in the NHS. The agency is to establish a national confidential incident reporting system that will include a facility to report diagnostic histopathology incidents or near misses. Incident reporting is an effective way of harnessing information that can be used to prevent future incidents and learn lessons for good practice. The success or failure of such systems depends on open and honest reporting by staff who know they will not be blamed individually for any adverse outcome. Anonymous and confidential error-reporting systems have a greater reporting rate compared to traditional reporting systems.[31] Incident reporting needs to include all errors, including near misses and staff need clear protocols and guidelines on the reporting process to encourage reporting of less serious incidents if lessons are to be learned.[32,33] When a serious incident has occurred, it is important that procedures and systems are in place to allow disclosure to be made to the patient by trained personnel; pathologists may need on occasion to be involved in this process. Laboratories and pathology services should ensure that systems are in place to report incidents systematically, trigger events and near misses. Organisational culture is important for learning from failures and should encourage reporting without blaming individuals when things go wrong. One of the basic principles of error management is that the best people can make the worst mistakes.

## HINDSIGHT BIAS

The 'knew it all along effect' is the universal tendency for humans to see past events as more foreseeable than they actually were. Those blessed with outcome knowledge see all the lines of causality homing in, but those equipped only with foresight do not always see this.[31] In the context of diagnostic histopathology, this is why retrospective reviews of slides are often biased and not a good measure of performance.

## CONCLUSIONS

The detection of errors and error avoidance in histopathology depends upon individuals practising to the highest standards by ensuring they are up-to-date and accountable for what they do. Pathologists should be willing to monitor their own performance, know their limitations and communicate with peers. Pathologists should engage in the process of developing standardised approaches to macroscopic description, specimen sampling, special stains and histological reporting. The laboratories in which they work should have in place systematised methods of audit, quality improvement and IT systems to support this and to identify poor performance at an early stage. The organisational culture should be blame-free and when things do go wrong, good risk management should be in place to prevent similar occurrences. A variety of methods can be used to detect errors in surgical pathology reporting. They provide quality assurance for patient diagnosis and are based on the explicit acceptance that histopathologists are not infallible while at the same time provide a useful way of detecting systematic sub-standard performance.

## Points of best practice

- The detection of errors and error avoidance in histopathology depends upon individuals practising to the highest standards by ensuring they are up-to-date and accountable for what they do.

- Pathologists should be willing to monitor their own performance, know their limitations and communicate with peers.

- Pathologists should engage in the process of developing standardised approaches to macroscopic description, specimen sampling, special stains and histological reporting.

- The laboratories in which pathologists work should have in place systematised methods of audit, quality improvement and IT systems to analyse the data and to identify poor performance at an early stage.

- The organisational culture should be blame-free and when things do go wrong, good risk management should be in place to prevent similar occurrences.

- A variety of methods can be used to detect errors in surgical pathology reporting. These provide quality assurance for patient diagnosis and are based on the explicit acceptance that histopathologists are not infallible while at the same time provide a useful way of detecting systematic sub-standard performance.

### References

1. Lesna M. Assessing diagnostic errors; when is suspension of a pathologist justified? *J Clin Pathol* 1998; **51**: 649–651.
2. Furness PN, Lauder I. A questionnaire based survey of errors in diagnostic histopathology throughout the UK. *J Clin Pathol* 1997; **50**: 457–460.
3. Ramsay AD. Errors in histopathology reporting: detection and avoidance. *Histopathology* 1999; **34**: 481–490.
4. Safrin RE, Bark CJ. Surgical pathology sign out; routine review of every case by a second pathologist. *Am J Surg Pathol* 1993; **17**: 1190–1192.
5. Lind AC, Bewtra C, Healy JC, Sims KL. Prospective peer review in surgical pathology. *Am J Clin Pathol* 1995; **104**: 560–566.
6. Stanley MW. Quality and liability issues with the Papanicolau smear; the role of professional organisations in reform initiatives. *Arch Pathol Lab Med* 1997; **121**: 327–330.
7. Ramsay AD, Gallagher PJ. Local audit of surgical pathology: 18 months' experience of peer review-based quality assessment in an English teaching hospital. *Am J Surg Pathol* 1992; **16**: 476–482.
8. Foucar E. Error identification; a surgical pathology dilemma. *Am J Surg Pathol* 1998; **22**; 1–5.
9. Poole CJM, Hill DJ, Christie JL, Birch J. Deficient colour vision and interpretation of histopathology slides: cross sectional study. *BMJ* 1997; **315**: 1279–1281.
10. Rigby HS, Warren BF, Diamond J, Carter C, Bradfield JWB Colour perception in pathologists: the Farnsworth-Munsell 100 hue test. *J Clin Pathol* 1991; **44**: 745–748.
11. Anon. *Learning from Bristol: The Report of the Public Inquiry into Children's Heart Surgery at the Bristol Royal Infirmary 1984–1995*. Bristol Royal Infirmary Inquiry, 2001.
12. Anon. *The Royal Liverpool Children's Inquiry: Summary and Recommendations*. London: Department of Health, 2001.

13. General Medical Council. *Good Medical Practice*. London: General Medical Council, 2001.

14. The Royal College of Pathologists. *Good Medical Practice in Pathology*. London: The Royal College of Pathologists, 2002.

15. The Royal College of Pathologists. *Substandard Professional Performance*. London: The Royal College of Pathologists, 2002.

16. Anon. Template for the assessment of professional performance in pathology specialties. *The Bulletin of the Royal College of Pathologists*, June 2002.

17. Rethans JJ, Norcini JJ, Baron-Maldonado M *et al*. The relationship between competence and performance: implications of assessing practice performance. *Med Educ* 2002; **36**: 901–909.

18. The Royal College of Pathologists. *Guidelines for the Appointment of Career Grade Locum Pathologists*. London: The Royal College of Pathologists, 2001.

19. Commission for Health Improvement. *Employing Locum Consultants – matters arising from the employment of Dr Elwood*. London: Commission for Health Improvement, 2001.

20. Arbiser ZK, Folpe AL, Weiss SW. Consultative (expert) second opinions in soft tissue pathology. Analysis of problem prone diagnostic situations. *Am J Surg Pathol* 2001; **116**: 473–476.

21. Parkes SE, Muir KR, Cameron AH *et al*. The need for specialist review of pathology in paediatric cancer. *Br J Cancer* 1997; **75**: 1156–1159.

22. 1st class service: quality in the NHS 1998.

23. Zardawi IM, Bennett G, Jain S, Brown M. Internal quality assurance activities of a surgical pathology department in an Australian teaching hospital. *J Clin Pathol* 1998; **51**: 695–699.

24. Wakeley SL, Baxendine-Jones JA, Gallagher, PJ, Mullee M, Pickering R. Aberrant diagnoses by individual surgical pathologists. *Am J Surg Pathol* 1997; **22**: 77–82.

25. Abt AB, Abt LG, Olt GJ. The effect of inter-institution anatomic pathology consultation on patient care. *Arch Pathol Lab Med* 1995; **119**: 514–517.

26. Renshaw AA, Pinnar NE, Jiroutek MR, Young ML. Quantifying the value of in-house consultation in surgical pathology. *Am J Clin Pathol* 2002; **117**: 751–754.

27. McBroom HM, Ramsay A. The clinico-pathological meeting. A means of auditing diagnostic performance. *Am J Surg Pathol* 1993; **17**: 75–80.

28. Nakhleh RE, Zaroo RJ. Amended reports in surgical pathology and implications for diagnostic error detection and avoidance: a College of American Pathologists' Q-probes study of 1,667,547 accessioned cases in 359 laboratories. *Arch Pathol Lab Med* 1998; **122**: 303–309.

29. Cross SS, Feeley KM, Angel CA. The effect of four interventions on the informational content of histopathology; reports of resected colonic carcinomas. *J Clin Pathol* 1998; **51**: 481–482.

30. Department of Health. *An Organisation with a Memory*. London: Stationery Office, 2000.

31. Reason J. Human error; models and management. *BMJ* 2000; **320**: 768–770.

32. Firth Cozens J. Barriers to incident reporting. *Qual Safety Health Care* 2002; **11**: 7.

33. Liang BA. A system of medical error disclosure. *Qual Safety Health Care* 2002; **11**: 64–68.

*Peter N. Furness*

8

# Ethical aspects of histopathology

Historically, histopathologists have paid little attention to problems of medical ethics but this has now changed. We have been made aware that patients and the relatives of a deceased person often expect the right to control what is done with their tissues, even small samples of tissue sent to the histopathology laboratory. This change was accelerated (but not initiated) in the UK by scandals over inappropriate retention of tissues after paediatric post mortems.[1–3] The public backlash to these revelations has had profound effects on many aspects of the practice of histopathology. Pathologists unfamiliar with ethical argument have found long-established procedures, which were believed to be good practice and intended to be for the benefit of patients, branded unethical. In some instances this condemnation is appropriate, but in others it represents the consequence of the 'politically correct' application of over-simplified rules by people who do not fully understand the consequences of these new restrictions.

As a result pathologists must now understand the relevant ethical arguments, not only to comply with good ethical practice in their routine work, but also to recognise inappropriate restrictions and mount philosophically sound arguments against them. This is a tall order for a specialty which has previously regarded issues such as consent to be the province of others. The aim of this short review is to provide some of the basic tools, vocabulary and arguments to facilitate the start of this transformation.

Of course, recognition of the importance of ethics in histopathological practice is not entirely new. The traditional ethical values of the medical profession are well recognised and have recently been set out in The Royal College of Pathologists' publication *Good Medical Practice in Pathology*. This document represents a pathology-specific supplement to the *Good Practice*

**Prof. Peter N. Furness** BM BCh PhD FRCPath
Professor of Renal Pathology, Division of Histopathology, Clinical Sciences Laboratories, Leicester General Hospital, Gwendolen Road, Leicester LE5 4PW, UK. Tel: +44 116 258 4582; Fax: 0116 258 4573
E-mail: peter.furness@le.ac.uk

series of publications by the General Medical Council. On the whole those issues are not recent advances. Much more relevant to this article is pathology's belated recognition of the shift in medical ethical thinking away from a 19th century paternalistic model towards one which respects and strives to enhance patient autonomy. It is this shift which has brought consent to the heart of current medical practice.

## INDIVIDUAL AUTONOMY – WHAT DOES IT MEAN?

The word autonomy is much used in medical ethics, but unfortunately it means different things to different people. It means self governance and was originally used to describe independent states rather than people. The concept of individual or personal autonomy was explored by the 19th century philosopher Immanuel Kant. Kant argued that humankind's capacities to consider the possible consequences of our actions, form intentions and act on them, rather than unreflectively reacting to circumstances, is what distinguishes us from machines and some (perhaps all) animals. This helps to define human beings as entities who deserve ethical consideration. Unthinking choices, for Kant, do not represent autonomy. For him, if an action is to be autonomous, rather than merely a reaction to subjective desires, the action is one which could, in theory, be adopted by all. (This 'universalisation' principle is known as the categorical imperative.) A decision to commit murder, theft or other obviously immoral act is not universalisable because if everyone acted in this way, society would break down. Similarly coercion, deception and the control or enslavement of others cannot be universally shared. The popular 'four principles' approach to medical ethics (respect for autonomy, beneficience, non-maleficience and justice[4]) can be derived on this basis.[5] This Kantian type of autonomy has been described as 'principled autonomy'.[6] Altruism is at the heart of Kantian free choice. It is easy to understand why the **principled** autonomy of individuals invariably deserves to be facilitated, respected and enhanced.

The need to enhance individual autonomy was promoted in the 1960s as one of four basic principles of medical ethics in a highly influential work by Beauchamp and Childress.[7] The other three were justice, beneficience and non-maleficience. Since then, respecting individual autonomy has come to be seen by many as the most important single principle. This emphasis on individual autonomy has driven the move away from 19th century paternalistic medical thinking. Patients must be empowered to make their own decisions about their healthcare. From this we derive the importance of valid, adequately informed consent in medical practice.

Most current argument in medical ethics uses a much simpler, libertarian concept of individual autonomy which can be explained simply as freedom of choice. Unfortunately, this shift eliminates the **universal** desirability of enhancing individual autonomy. This is rarely noticed in medical ethics, where patients are usually making decisions which are for their own benefit and which do not affect others, but the distinction is very obvious in most other walks of life. Most of the criminal law is about limiting this libertarian type of individual autonomy. If a person autonomously decides to murder, steal, fail to pay taxes or drive dangerously then facilitating such 'libertarian autonomous' acts clearly cannot be supported. Environmental ethics is largely about **limiting** individual free choice in order to preserve the ecosystem. There is an obvious need to balance the enhancement of **libertarian** individual autonomy against the needs of society or 'the good of all'.

The current concerns about the uses of human tissue show a degree of inconsistency here. To run a modern health service such as the NHS requires money. It also requires human tissue for teaching, quality control and research. If citizens who expect to benefit from the NHS exercise their libertarian autonomy by deciding not to pay taxes, they will feel the full weight of the law. If libertarian autonomy is exercised by insisting that excised tissue is incinerated instead of being used for the good of all, society regards that decision as entirely acceptable. Neither act represents autonomy in the Kantian sense, as neither is universalisable.

## WHAT IS CONSENT?

The requirements of consent have been recently set out by the UK Department of Health.[8] They include:

- *The provision of adequate information*
- *A capacity to understand that information*
- *Time to consider the questions involved, at least as far as practical*
- *An absence of coercion.*

These requirements raise several problems. Problems with the capacity to understand (children, the unconscious, the mentally ill or those who are just physically ill) have been considered elsewhere.[8] At times there is no alternative but to fall back on carefully considered paternalism, but this must be avoided wherever possible. 'Adequate' information must include the range of choices which are possible, together with the possible outcomes of each choice and some estimate of the probability of each. This of course means that a request to use surplus tissue for teaching or research is not adequately informed unless the patient is aware that the usual alternative is for it to be incinerated as clinical waste. 'Fully informed consent' is a commonly used but meaningless term; to know absolutely everything about anything is a logical impossibility. 'Adequately', 'sufficiently' or 'appropriately' recognises this, and also implies the need to consider what is adequate, sufficient and appropriate. However, decisions may be required on the extent to which extremely rare outcomes or complications need to be discussed. There are different types of consent. The following terms will be used.

1. **Explicit consent** (sometimes called express consent) means that the issues have been explicitly discussed with the patient and an explicit decision has been expressed by the patient. This is commonly followed by a signature on a consent form, though it is important to recognise that the signature and the form do not themselves represent 'consent', nor do they prove the existence of valid consent – they merely provide some evidence to suggest that an appropriate consent process has occurred.

2. **Implied consent** is very widely used for minor procedures in medicine. In an appropriate context, holding out an arm implies consent to venepuncture; consulting a doctor implies consent for the doctor to read the medical records. The

action of the patient implies consent to the logical subsequent action of the doctor. In its most robust form, inaction cannot imply consent. Under this robust definition, merely providing information (such as posting an information leaflet) does not imply consent unless the recipient demonstrates in some way that the information has been received (*e.g.* by attending an out-patient's appointment which was provided with the information leaflet).[9]

3. **Specific consent** relates to a set of circumstances which is closely defined in the information which has been provided. An example might be consent to use tissues in a single research project or on one occasion.

4. **General (or generic) consent** implies wider permission, such as consent to use tissue for any type of medical training. If general consent is to be valid, one must ask whether the information provided was adequate; were all possible consequences for the patient appropriately explained? In the context of histopathology, this usually means that general consent is appropriate only where there can be no adverse consequences for the patient. Hence, if 'general consent for research use' of tissues is to be acceptable, it is essential that there should be zero risk of any specific adverse consequences for the patient. To take an extreme example, testing named samples for a genetic predisposition for a fatal, untreatable neurodegenerative disorder would be completely unacceptable on the basis of 'general consent to research use', because the patient has not had the opportunity to consider the possible adverse consequences of such information becoming available.

These types of consent are often regarded as having different value; for example, explicit consent is 'better' than implied consent. In relation to the *Data Protection Act 1998*, the Information Commissioner has stated:

> It is a mistake to assume that implied consent is a less valid form of consent than express. Both must be equally informed and both reflect the wishes of the patient. The advantage of express consent is that it is less likely to be ambiguous and may thus be preferred when the risk of misunderstanding is greater.[9]

It should be recognised that in suitable circumstances they all may satisfy the necessary criteria for adequate, valid consent.

## IS CONSENT SUFFICIENT?

Consent is not a licence to do absolutely anything. In medical practice, consent does not make an invasive procedure ethically acceptable if that procedure has no prospect of therapeutic benefit. Similarly, consent to use tissue for unethical purposes does not make such use acceptable. The Nuffield Council on Bioethics has provided an excellent analysis of what constitutes ethical use of human tissue. The arguments remain compelling despite recent changes in what is regarded as valid consent.[10]

## THE RELEVANCE OF CONSENT IN DIAGNOSTIC HISTOPATHOLOGY PRACTICE

The responsible clinician should have obtained the patient's consent to take a sample. For some samples (urine, faeces, blood), consent may be implied and there will be no signature on a consent form. This does not mean that consent has not been obtained, merely that it has not been documented. Solid tissue samples should invariably be obtained after formal explicit consent. However, the consent form is likely to relate to the procedure of removing the sample rather than consent for examination of the sample. Nevertheless, when a biopsy is taken specifically for diagnosis the pathologist can reasonably infer that consent is available for investigation. (If not, then the biopsy serves no purpose, in which case taking the biopsy represents ethically unjustifiable mutilation, even if the patient has signed a consent form).

The situation is slightly less clear in relation to major surgical resections. The clinical team will invariably gain consent for the surgical procedure, but the pathologist can rarely be certain that consent to subsequent pathological examination has also been obtained. To assume such consent is normal practice, but may be viewed by some as paternalistic. It is quite possible that the patient may see the removal of the abnormal tissue as the only purpose of the procedure. In this situation, if we believe the patient retains the right to control what happens to the tissue, it is arguable that consent does not necessarily extend to histological examination. The same argument applies to disposal of the tissue; but here, 'do nothing' is not an option. In practice, most pathologists (consciously or subconsciously) either assume that this is a problem for the clinical team or that histological examination is justified because it is in the patients' best interest. The former can be seen as an abdication of professional duty; the latter as a lapse into the paternalism which has caused our profession so much trouble in the past. This is an area which has so far escaped critical attention, perhaps because the vast majority of patients are actually completely unconcerned about what happens to resected 'surgical waste',[11] and the few who are concerned make their wishes known. Nevertheless, this argument makes it clear that if a patient actively objects to histological examination of resected tissue, or wishes to have that tissue returned, then (subject to health and safety considerations) we should as far as possible comply with such demands after having done our best to explain the possible consequences.

This discussion so far relates to primary histological diagnosis. Histopathologists are usually obliged to assume (correctly or not) that the referring clinician has discussed the likely outcome of the histological examination with the patient. If this has been done properly it would include the possibility of a completely unsuspected diagnosis being made. When histological examination leads to the suspicion of such a diagnosis, it is generally considered good clinical practice to carry out what clinical chemists refer to as 'reflex testing' – further investigations to prove or disprove the new hypothesis. These would typically include immunohistochemistry or special stains (*e.g.* a Ziehl Neelsen stain to confirm tuberculosis), or more recently PCR identification of a microbial genome. In most circumstances, to seek renewed patient consent for such investigations would seem absurd. We assume the patient wants the correct diagnosis. To seek renewed consent would cause delay, consume resources, probably annoy the patient and potentially damage clinical care. However, this assumption of consent for further investigation is arguably another example of paternalism. In at least one situation it is unequivocally not permissible – AIDS. If histological appearances lead to a suspicion of HIV infection, it is generally accepted that explicit, specific consent is required before a confirmatory test can be performed. HIV is an extreme example, but there are undoubtedly other diagnoses which adequately informed patients may decide that they do not wish to know. The potential for 'reflex testing' to cause objections and even litigation is clear, and pathologists should remain aware of this potential problem, especially as new laboratory investigations move into clinical practice.

## WHAT HAPPENS TO TISSUE AFTER EXAMINATION?

When histopathological examination is complete, the remaining tissue could be stored, disposed of, returned to the patient or used for some socially and ethically acceptable purpose (*i.e.* for the benefit of all). Here, decisions might appear to relate to 'ownership' of the tissue, except that current UK legislation does not permit the ownership of body parts. Case law has in the past suggested that if tissues are 'substantially modified' then the person who exercised the skill of modification generates for themselves some form of ownership. (Regina *v* Kelly) However, in the present climate this seems unlikely to be accepted and the current review of UK legislation[12] is likely to conclude that patients should be empowered to control what happens to their tissues under almost all circumstances. We have recently seen a revolution whereby any tissue retained at post mortem must now be accompanied by detailed information about consent for further use and disposal. This is not so in relation to therapeutic removal of tissue from the living. The discrepancy is perhaps justified by the clear differences in the emotional importance of post mortem tissue when compared to 'surgical waste'.[11,13] Nevertheless, if we are to avoid paternalism (and vigorous objections from a minority of patients), we need to know the wishes of the patients. How might this be achieved?

### DISPOSAL OR STORAGE

Current practice in most hospitals is that surplus tissue resected from the living is incinerated. Patients are very rarely consulted about this. When they are consulted, most raise no objection[11,13] and in most circumstances it is unlikely that issues such as the definition of 'respectful disposal' have the importance they assume with post mortem tissue. A few samples do have greater emotional significance. Products of conception, eyes, whole limbs and resected sexual organs represent likely examples. Here it is particularly inappropriate and paternalistic to assume that incineration as clinical waste will be acceptable to the patient. Of course, alternatives such as returning the specimen to the patient raise significant health and safety problems. It is perfectly possible that the patient might want to obtain resected tissue for purposes which society might consider distasteful or even ethically unacceptable. Nonetheless, few would argue that we should not at least try to comply with the wishes of patients where these are expressed. In practice, such requests are extremely rare. This either implies that patients are rarely asked to consider the ultimate fate of resected tissue, or that almost all are unconcerned what it is. Probably both – but how can we find out?

# TEACHING, QUALITY ASSURANCE AND RESEARCH

These are all areas where, to run a modern health service, it is necessary to use human tissue for 'the common good'. Therefore, there is potential for conflict between the wishes of an individual and the needs of society. There is a degree of inconsistency in the ways in which this balance is decided. For example, when society deems it necessary to ascertain a cause of death, the Coroner is empowered to order a post mortem examination, with retention and examination of tissues, even if this is clearly contrary to deeply held religious views of the patient and relatives. Here, the needs of society over-ride individual concerns. One might reasonably suggest that saving life is of greater importance to society than ascertaining a cause of death; but when organs are needed for transplantation, a single objection from one relative will over-ride the prospect of saving another's life, with its consequent benefit for society.[14]

The development of modern healthcare services could not have occurred without human tissues having been used in research, and can not be maintained without on-going use of human tissues for teaching and quality assurance. If we apply the Kantian 'categorical imperative', we might suggest that if a patient refuses to allow such use of surgical waste, while still expecting to use modern healthcare, the patient is acting immorally, because the action is not 'universalisable'. If everyone refused, the health services could not exist in their present form.

Most commentators fall back upon the simpler, libertarian definition of autonomy rather than Kantian 'principled autonomy' as discussed above. This has almost universally been interpreted as indicating that consent is required for such activities. We should not make the mistake of believing that this is some basic inviolable right, rather that it is a right which society chooses to provide, and can do so only because of the generosity of the majority of people who give consent. If everyone refused consent, society would be obliged to apply enforcement procedures, just as with the Coroner's rules, or with the early Anatomy Acts which sought to guarantee a supply of cadavers for the advancement of medical research.

## TEACHING AND QUALITY ASSURANCE

It is generally assumed that patient consent is not needed for 'apprenticeship' training where junior pathologists examine histological sections before confirmation of the diagnosis by a senior member of staff. For a patient to refuse consent for such work would be tantamount to demanding medical care exclusively from a senior consultant and nursing care from the ward sister. Such demands could not be accommodated so consent is unnecessary: whether explicitly discussed or not, compliance is a precondition of the provision of healthcare. Recent Department of Health advice[8] indicates that for other aspects of teaching and quality control consent is required but implied, generic consent is deemed to be acceptable. Patient confidentiality must be preserved, usually by anonymisation of the sample. NHS hospitals are now required to inform patients that surplus tissues may be used for these purposes and to invite patients who object to make their views known.

This has highlighted a problem which legislators have so far largely ignored. Obtaining consent, or recording objections, is not sufficient; there has to be a mechanism by which the existence of consent or objection can be checked by those who need to use the tissues. At the time of writing, despite central insistence on the importance of implied consent,[8] few hospitals have made progress in implementing the necessary infrastructure to provide laboratory staff with a practical procedure by which the presence or absence of consent or objection can be checked before every single use of human tissue. If there is no mechanism by which to act on the decision of the patient, then the consent process is a sham.

This new requirement, to inform patients of how tissues may be used, has close similarities to recent advice from the Information Commissioner on the implementation of the *Data Protection Act 1998* in relation to medical information. The Information Commissioner demands that 'fair processing information' be provided to all patients, informing them of how their personal data may be used by the health service, and inviting objections.[9] It would appear to possible to satisfy both these requirements with a single procedure, but so far little progress has been made.

The UK Government has indicated that consent for using tissue in teaching and quality control should be implied and generic.[8] If generic consent is to be acceptable, then the specific uses covered by this consent must be non-controversial and must have no potential for adverse impact on the patients' interests. For use in teaching, if confidentiality is adequately maintained this is surely the case. If risks to the patient existed they would have to have been discussed, or the consent would be inadequately informed and hence invalid; if there are known specific risks, then the consent must also be specific.

Initial advice from the General Medical Council suggested that the publication of images derived from **any** patient-based material would require explicit consent, even if there were no way in which the patient concerned could recognise the material as being his or her own. This requirement would cause considerable difficulty for the publication of educational material in histopathology. When clinical photographs are taken, the patient is present and consent can easily be requested. The same is not true when a photograph is taken from a microscope slide. Fortunately, the General Medical Council has recently revised this view, and explicit consent is no longer deemed necessary for the publication of suitably anonymised photomicrographs.[15]

## RESEARCH

It is in the area of using surplus human tissue in research projects where histopathologists have perhaps encountered the most perplexing ethical dilemmas. In the past, histopathologists generally regarded the pathology archive as a resource which could be legitimately used for medical research for the good of all without patient consent, bearing in mind the need to preserve confidentiality. This view was supported by a detailed ethical review published in 1995 which concluded that surgically resected tissues could be regarded as 'abandoned' by the patient unless specific instructions to the contrary were given.[10]

This position has been radically amended since publication of the paediatric autopsy tissue retention scandals,[1,2] despite the different emotional importance of post mortem tissue and surgical waste discussed above. Research which uses human tissue (or biological fluids) must first be approved by an appropriate research ethics committee (REC).[16,17] Consent is now deemed essential for the research use of 'surplus' human tissue. General 'consent for research use' is probably acceptable as long as the research poses no prospect of harming the tissue donors' best interests and is in a non-controversial area. ('Non-controversial' excludes not only obvious areas such as developing weapons of biological warfare, but also less obvious areas such as research into contraception, where it is foreseeable that some religious groups would object.)

## WHAT SORT OF CONSENT?

An analogy with teaching and quality control might suggest that implied consent should be sufficient for some research projects, where (as with teaching and quality control) it is inconceivable that the data generated could have an adverse impact on the patient, the work is non-controversial and is 'for the common good'. However, current UK Department of Health guidance suggests that 'valid' consent will usually be a requirement for research use of human tissue.[17] Most RECs have interpreted this as meaning explicit consent, with a signature on a consent form. While this is understandable for some forms of research, it seems difficult to justify as a blanket requirement for any logical reason beyond a general mistrust of science. Guidance from the Medical Research Council (MRC)[16] and the Department of Health[17] indicates that there may be some circumstances where research using archival samples is permissible without consent, such as when re-contacting the tissue donor may cause distress or when re-contacting the donor is impractical. Unfortunately, many RECs have been reluctant to allow the use of these clauses.

## PATIENTS SHOULD CONTROL THEIR TISSUES: TWO LOGICAL CONSEQUENCES, NOT ONE

The basic argument, which I believe we should accept without hesitation, is that patients must be empowered to control what happens to their tissue. We must conclude from this that is it immoral to use tissue against the wishes of the patient. To do so may be called 'the sin of the researcher'. But this is only half of the conclusion. Logically, the other half is that it is immoral to **prohibit** the use of tissue for the good of all if that is what the patient wants. Even if the patient is completely apathetic, then surely the prospect of benefit to medical science should carry the decision. Inappropriate prohibition may be described as 'the sin of the regulator'.

Unethical prohibition, 'the sin of the regulator', is considered irrelevant by many commentators, who would say that if you obtain consent, the problem is solved – it becomes clear what may and may not be done. Those directly involved in this type of work will recognise the problem here – the difficulty of obtaining consent. Even if we ignore issues of time and resources, laboratory workers often have no access to patients and busy clinicians are often not inclined to help. Some of the patients may have died, and if the deceased are automatically included in (or excluded from) the study, the resultant patient sample is biased. With archival samples, patients or their relatives may object to being reminded about episodes of illness from long ago.

The problem of obtaining consent for the use of archival samples has been considered by the MRC and the UK Department of Health. It may, for example, be unethical to re-contact cancer patients years after they consider themselves 'cured', because to do so may raise fears of recurrence in their minds and so cause distress. This is obviously a difficult decision to make and RECs can be expected to vary in its application. It can also be difficult to decide when it is 'impractical' to obtain consent. We recently undertook to seek explicit, generic consent from all Leicestershire's renal transplant patients for research use of archived tissue and data. This should be an ideal group for this exercise; the population is stable and the patients are never discharged. An initial letter requesting consent was followed up by tracing in the out-patient clinics those who did not reply. Despite all this work, one year after the project started we still do not know the wishes of 26% of the patients. Less than 3% have objected, so if we now run a project where explicit consent is required, it is likely that 25% of patients will be excluded from the project against their wishes. In recent years ethics committees have been far more concerned with avoiding the use of tissues against the wishes of the patient than they have been with avoiding the prohibition of use against the wishes of the patient. The difficulty of obtaining consent in this context has been underestimated and as a consequence many research projects have been blocked. In this situation, evidence that it is impractical to obtain consent comes too late.

## REMOVING TISSUE PRIOR TO PATHOLOGICAL EXAMINATION

It is common for research projects to require fresh tissue, necessitating removal before the specimen has been examined in the histopathology laboratory. This is usually considered to be a special case. Specific explicit consent from the patient is almost invariably required with a signature on a specifically designed consent form. It is debatable whether this requirement is logical. Although sometimes neglected, the main point is surely that the removal of tissue must not compromise the subsequent histopathological examination. If it does, then the patient has been harmed, and the fact that consent has been obtained does not make the procedure ethical. On the other hand, if the removal does not affect the subsequent pathological examination, it is difficult to see why procedures should be different from removing tissue after the pathological examination is complete. From the patient's viewpoint the effect is indistinguishable. The crucial point is that pathological examination should not be compromised. The requirement for 'extra' consent procedures is, therefore, not an ethical issue but a risk management issue, introduced just in case pathological examination is compromised. But this is futile, because if examination is compromised, the 'extra' consent is worthless.

It follows that whenever tissues are removed for research before pathological examination, there should be an agreement between clinician, researcher and pathology laboratory to ensure an adequate exchange of information which will safeguard the pathological examination.

## 'THE *HELICOBACTER* TEST': A TEST FOR NEW LEGISLATION?

In contemplating how to resolve these problems, and hence the balance between individual rights and the good of all, it is instructive to consider how regulations might have affected the discovery of Helicobacter pylori as the causative agent of gastritis and peptic ulceration. Under current requirements, to follow-up the initial observation of curved structures resembling bacteria in H&E sections of gastric biopsies,[18] a histopathologist would have to obtain REC approval and probably explicit consent from all patients concerned. This would apply even to reviewing slides from the archive, which in this context is unquestionably 'research'. Under these circumstances, it seems very unlikely that a busy histopathologist would be inclined to follow-up the initial chance observation; so the current guidance fails 'the *Helicobacter* test'. The result would be that we would still be treating peptic ulceration with major abdominal operations rather than antibiotics. In the current ethical debate in this area, it seems customary to pay lip service to the potential benefits of research to mankind, but this concrete example demonstrates how restrictions imposed apparently to enhance individual autonomy can inadvertently cause widespread damage to the very individuals the regulations are trying to protect.

How can we avoid the sin of the researcher and the sin of the regulator? Only by knowing the wishes of all patients. This argument was behind recent proposals from The Royal College of Pathologists,[19] which suggested that initially research using surplus tissue should be permissible under implied consent, as is now accepted for teaching. We should rapidly move to a system where every patient's views are recorded explicitly. Such a system could resolve many other issues, such as consent to organ donation, autopsy and post mortem tissue retention, advance directives and so on. It would enhance individual autonomy and relieve relatives of agonising decisions at times of great distress. It would also be expensive and at the time of writing such a system seems unlikely to be implemented.

## SO WHAT DO RESEARCH ETHICS COMMITTEES WANT?

At present, this question cannot be answered because different RECs are imposing radically different requirements. They have suddenly been asked to review tissue-based research projects which were previously outside their remit. Their membership rarely includes histopathologists but commonly includes people who have been understandably alarmed by tissue retention scandals and may see their role as preventing any further controversy. The committee will be familiar with considering clinical trials, in which direct patient contact is inevitable, so the difficulties experienced by laboratory workers who are told to obtain consent are not understood. Prohibition of research or the imposition of further requirements is not seen as controversial (despite the '*Helicobacter* test' described above). Furthermore, the situation has been muddied by the publication of several sets of guidelines, some of which do not consider post mortem tissue and 'surgical waste' separately. To avoid controversy, there is a tendency to extract the most restrictive elements from all the guidelines and apply them all, sometimes with additional restrictions just for good measure. For example, some RECs have not allowed patients to consent to assist with any research, limiting consent to research into the disease from which the patient is suffering. This not only blocks altruism, it also (very unfashionably) limits patient autonomy. Sadly, until attitudes change it seems inevitable that pathologists will be frustrated when applying for approval of tissue-based research projects. To minimise the frustration, the following steps are recommended.

- Read carefully a single, appropriate and authoritative source of guidance, preferably one recommended by the REC

- It is not sufficient merely to comply with this guidance – you must prove that you are complying by extensive references to specific points of guidance. Do not assume that the committees know the details of such guidance: at least one ethics committee referred a researcher to the MRC guidance while simultaneously making a comment which displayed ignorance of its contents. Be wary of locally produced guidelines; ask how they were derived, as they may add extra layers to the national guidance they purport to follow

- Demonstrate explicitly your understanding of the importance of consent, individual autonomy and confidentiality

- Not only design the experiment to uphold these principles, but explain, in detail and as often as possible, how you have done so. If you are unable to obtain the explicit, specific consent of every patient involved, do not merely say so: explain why, and how failing to carry out the project would be a greater disservice to the patients and to society than not obtaining such consent

- The REC is likely to demand patient consent of some type for most projects. The MRC guidelines make it plain that consent is not invariably needed for all tissue-based research. Unfortunately, this decision depends on subjective evaluations of the benefit of the research to society, the potential for any adverse impact on the patient and the difficulty which obtaining consent would incur. These features all need to be explained carefully. Some RECs still assume that any attempt to suggest that consent should not be sought represents a researcher who is trying to complicate matters in order to avoid doing the necessary work

- This need for detailed explanation is not helped by mandatory REC application forms – it will often be necessary to include a covering letter to explain these points adequately.

## CONCLUSIONS

Many histopathologists will conclude that these new restrictions, especially in relation to research, are excessive, bureaucratic, wasteful of resources and contrary to the common good. They fail 'the *Helicobacter* test'. In many respects this view is justified, but histopathologists operate within the confines of society and we must accept that society is increasingly suspicious of 'science', 'experts', and (since the tissue retention scandals) especially pathologists. The importance of individual autonomy as a concept in medical ethics is here to stay. Pathologists who wish to operate at maximal efficiency for the benefit of all will need to understand the arguments and make their case repeatedly and forcefully in the future.

## ACKNOWLEDGEMENT

I am grateful to my wife Dr S.H. Furness for her assistance with my attempt to explain the philosophical background of the concept of individual autonomy.

---

### Points for best practice

- Modern medical ethics places emphasis on enhancing patient autonomy.

- Respect for autonomy means that pathologists must avoid paternalism and consider whether they have the patient's consent for their work.

- There are differing views of autonomy. If autonomy is taken to mean simply freedom of choice it may ignore any responsibility to society. In life outside medical ethics, devices to ensure responsible behaviour curtail this over-simplified notion of autonomy.

- A violent reaction against work carried out without genuine consent has led to severe restrictions on how pathologists work. Although applied with good intentions, some of these are clearly contrary to the interests of society.

- If pathologists are to operate efficiently they will in future be obliged to engage in ethical arguments, balancing the rights of individuals against the rights of society. This requires greater understanding of basic ethical and philosophical principles.

---

### References

1. *The Inquiry into the Management of Care of Children receiving Complex Heart Surgery at the Bristol Royal Infirmary.* 2000. <http://www.bristol-inquiry.org.uk/>.
2. *The Report of The Royal Liverpool Children's Inquiry* (the 'Richards Report'). 2001. <http://www.rlcinquiry.org.uk/>.
3. *Report of a Census of Organs and Tissues Retained by Pathology Services in England.* 2001. <http://www.doh.gov.uk/organcensus/>.
4. Beauchamp T. The 'four-principles' approach. In: Gillon R. (ed) *Principles of Health Care Ethics.* Chichester: Wiley, 1994; 4–12.
5. Furness SH. Medical ethics, Kant and mortality. In: Gillon R. (ed) *Principles of Health Care Ethics.* Chichester: Wiley, 1994; 159–171.
6. O'Neill O. *Autonomy and Trust in Bioethics.* Cambridge: Cambridge University Press, 2002.
7. Beauchamp T, Childress J. *Principles of Biomedical Ethics,* 3rd edn. New York: Oxford University Press, 1989.
8. Department of Health. *Good Practice in Consent Implementation Guide: Consent to Examination or Treatment.* London: HMSO, 2001. <http://www.doh.gov.uk/consent/implementationguide.pdf>.

9. Office of the Information Commissioner, UK Government. *Use and Disclosure of Health Data: Guidance on the Application of the Data Protection Act 1998.* 2002. <http://www.dataprotection.gov.uk/dpr/dpdoc.nsf>.

10. Nuffield Council on Bioethics. *Human Tissue: Ethical and Legal Issues.* London: The Nuffield Foundation, 1995 <http://www.nuffieldfoundation.org/bioethics/>.

11. Medical Research Council. *Public Perceptions of the Collection of Human Biological Samples.* London: MRC, 2001 <http://www.wellcome.ac.uk/en/images/biolcoll_3182.pdf>.

12. Department of Health. *Review of the Law relating to Human Organs and Tissue.* London: HMSO, 2002 <http://www.doh.gov.uk/tissue/review_of_law.htm>.

13. Start RD, Brown W, Bryant RJ *et al.* Ownership and uses of human tissue: does the Nuffield bioethics report accord with opinion of surgical inpatients? *BMJ* 1996; **313**: 1366–1368.

14. Department of Health. *Human Bodies, Human Choices. The law on human organs and tissue in England and Wales. A consultation report.* London: HMSO, 2002 <http://www.doh.gov.uk/tissue/choices.pdf>.

15. General Medical Council. *Making and Using Visual and Audio Recordings of Patients.* London: GMC, 2002 <http://www.gmc-uk.org/standards/aud_vid.htm>.

16. Medical Research Council. *Human Tissue and Biological Samples for use in Research: Operational and Ethical Guidelines.* London: MRC, 2001 <http://www.mrc.ac.uk/pdf-tissue_guide_fin.pdf>.

17. Department of Health, UK Government. *An interim statement on the use of human organs and tissue.* London, HMSO, 2003. http://www.doh.gov.uk/tissue/interimstatement.htm

18. Marshall BJ, Warren JR. Unidentified curved bacilli in the stomach of patients with gastritis and peptic ulceration. *Lancet* 1984; **1**: 1311–1315.

19. The Royal College of Pathologists. *Transitional guidelines to facilitate changes in procedures for handling 'surplus' and archival material from human biological samples.* London: The Royal College of Pathologists, 2001 <http://www.rcpath.org/transition.html>.

*S.B. Wharton, M.S. Fernando, P.G. Ince*

**9**

# Neuropathology of hypoxia

Hypoxia is a broad term that may encompass states of inadequate delivery or utilisation of oxygen such that tissue and cell function are compromised. This review will focus on the brain, in which hypoxia may contribute to a number of pathological states. In ambient air, with a $PO_2$ of 21 kPa, arterial $PO_2$ is 12–15 kPa (90–110 mmHg). Within the brain the tissue $PO_2$ is low, falling to values of around 4 kPa, but this varies from region to region and with brain activity. The tissue $PO_2$ correlates with blood flow so that, under normal circumstances, cerebral blood flow and oxygen consumption are coupled.[1] The high energy requirements of cerebral tissue for maintaining ion gradients and intracellular transport within neurons and their dependence on aerobic metabolism render the brain very vulnerable to the interruption of oxygen supply.

In terms of causation, hypoxia is classically divided into hypoxic, stagnant (hypoxic-ischaemic) and histotoxic types.[2] Of these, the pathologist is most commonly called upon to assess the hypoxic-ischaemic type. Hypoxia is only one component of ischaemia; the two are not equivalent and, as will be discussed, the effects of hypoxia and ischaemia on the brain differ. In addition to these classical types of hypoxic brain disorder, there is an increasing appreciation that hypoxia and hypoxic cellular response mechanisms play a role in many CNS disorders including neurodegenerative diseases and neoplasms.

This review will discuss: (i) the neuropathology of hypoxic and global hypoxia-ischaemic states; (ii) aspects of the pathways by which cells die in

**Dr S.B. Wharton** BSc MBBS MSc MRCPath
Senior Clinical Lecturer in Neuropathology, Academic Unit of Pathology, University of Sheffield, Medical School, Beech Hill Road, Sheffield S10 2RX, UK
Tel: +44 114 271 2683; Fax: +44 114 226 1464; E-mail: s.wharton@sheffield.ac.uk (for correspondence)

**Dr M.S. Fernando** MBBS Dip Pathol, MD (Histopath)
Academic Commonwealth Scholar (as above)

**Professor P.G. Ince** BSc MBBS MD FRCPath
Professor of Neuropathology (as above)

129

hypoxia-ischaemia; (iii) recent advances in the cellular response to hypoxia, focusing particularly on the roles of neuroglobin and of hypoxia-inducible factor; and (iv) evidence of a role for hypoxia and for hypoxia-responsive elements in a variety of CNS disorders.

## PURE HYPOXIC STATES

Isolated impairment of oxygen supply, without accompanying circulatory compromise (leading to ischaemia) is uncommon. It may occur clinically, for example, in young children with respiratory obstruction. The brain is sensitive to oxygen deprivation and cells deprived of oxygen will die if oxygenation is not restored.[1] *In vivo*, the pure hypoxic state differs from ischaemia – ischaemia involves a failure of delivery of other substrates and of removal of waste products such as lactate and $CO_2$ resulting in tissue acidosis.[2] Good clinical recovery has been reported after hypoxic coma with little residual neurological deficit, in contrast to the effects of global hypoxic-ischaemic coma.[3,4] In rare cases where patients have died suddenly after prolonged respiratory hypoxia with maintained perfusion, little neuropathology has been found.[5] In experimental models, hypoxia exacerbates the effects of ischaemia, but alone appears to produce little necrosis or changes in tissue levels of glutamate.[6,7] Hypoxia as an isolated event appears, therefore, to cause less tissue damage than when it is accompanied by a deficit in perfusion.

## HYPOXIC-ISCHAEMIC ENCEPHALOPATHY

### NEUROPATHOLOGY

Whilst focal ischaemia occurs in the context of stroke, this section will focus on the pathology of transient global hypoxia-ischaemia. Some authors prefer not to include 'hypoxia' in the terminology, given that it is the ischaemia with impairment of perfusion rather than hypoxia *per se* that appears to be the more significant. Certainly the term 'stagnant hypoxia' is no longer useful as it fails to convey the key pathogenetic concepts. Global hypoxic-ischaemic events are associated with general circulatory collapse, classically seen in encephalopathy after cardiac arrest and as a component of shock states. The effects on the brain may be widespread and vary from case to case. In general terms, the distribution of damage is determined by the vascular anatomy of the brain and by the degree of vulnerability of particular cell types. The severity of disease may be modified by factors such as the duration and degree of ischaemia, pre-existing vascular disease, blood glucose, age of the patient, and body temperature – hypothermia is protective.[2,8]

Neurons are more susceptible to hypoxic-ischaemic insult than glia and so may be selectively affected in a transient event. A more severe or sustained insult will result in necrosis of all components producing infarction. Transient global hypoxia-ischaemia characteristically affects certain vulnerable neuronal groups. In adults, the hippocampus is commonly affected, especially the pyramidal neurons of the CA1 (Sommer's sector) and CA4 (end-folium) regions (Fig. 1). In the cerebral cortex, neurons in layers 3, 5 and 6 have particular vulnerability which produces a laminar pattern of damage. Areas of

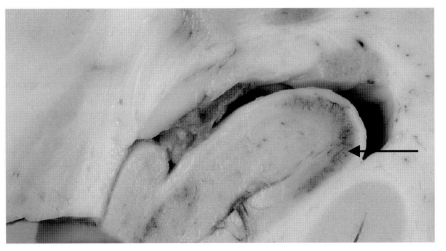

**Fig. 1** Hippocampus showing discolouration of the CA1 region (arrow) due to hypoxic-ischaemic injury.

cortex in the sulci are more vulnerable than over the crests of gyri. Neurons within the basal ganglia, particularly the lateral striatum, and the Purkinje cells of the cerebellum are also especially vulnerable. In addition to the intrinsic vulnerability of particular neuronal groups, the boundary zones between vascular territories are susceptible as they are areas in which cerebral blood flow is at its most precarious. These areas include: (i) the anterior and middle cerebral artery boundary zone in the parasaggital cortex; (ii) the triple watershed area between the anterior, middle and posterior cerebral arteries in the occipital cortex; and (iii) the boundary between the territories of the superior and inferior cerebellar arteries in the cerebellum.[8–10] Recent hypoxic-ischaemic damage can be recognised macroscopically by patchy discolouration. In patients who survive for several months, the brain is reduced in weight with cortical atrophy and enlarged ventricles. Examination of the cortex may reveal laminar cavitation and the hippocampi may be small and sclerotic.[11]

## EFFECTS ON NEURONS

After an acute hypoxic-ischaemic insult, neurons may show ischaemic neuronal change (Fig. 2). This histological appearance may be seen with survival intervals of about 6 h and represents developing neuronal death. Neurons show shrinkage of the soma and increasing eosinophilia of the cytoplasm. The nucleus also shrinks, taking on a more darkly stained, triangular appearance.[9] Care should be taken not to mis-interpret the presence of neurons with darkly stained (rather than eosinophilic) cytoplasm that often have dendrites with a corkscrew appearance: the distribution of these cells does not correlate with areas of vulnerability and this appearance of dark cell change is probably artefactual. There is evidence from careful pathological studies of human material that, in comparison with cortical areas, neuronal damage in the hippocampus may be delayed.[12] The concept of delayed neuronal death, which is supported by experimental studies, implies that certain neurons do not die immediately after a hypoxic-ischaemic insult, but do so because of initiation of processes operative in the post-ischaemic period.[2] The dissection of the relevant molecular events in hypoxic-ischaemic cell injury may offer a potential therapeutic window. The pathologist should also be aware in the assessment of a case that the appearance of some morphological changes may be delayed after the injurious event.

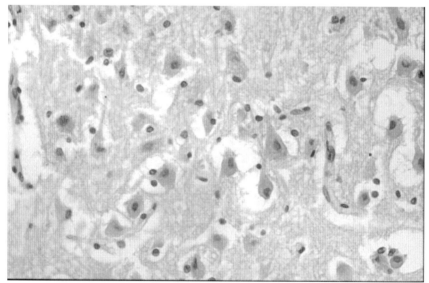

**Fig. 2** Pyramidal neurons within the CA1 region of the hippocampus showing acute hypoxic-ischaemic neuronal cell change. The cells are shrunken with a more homogeneous cytoplasm which, with conventional stains, appears eosinophilic. The nuclei are also shrunken, more darkly stained and somewhat triangular in shape.

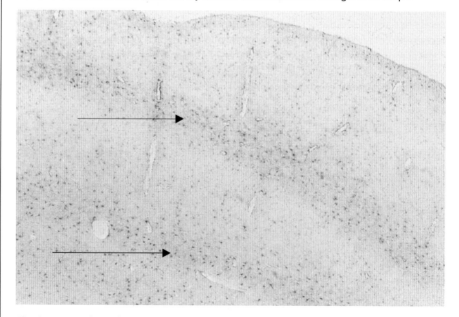

**Fig. 3** Immunohistochemistry to GFAP showing a laminar pattern of gliosis in the cerebral cortex. The gliosis forms two bands (arrows), representing a glial reaction to selective neuronal injury in layers 3 and 5.

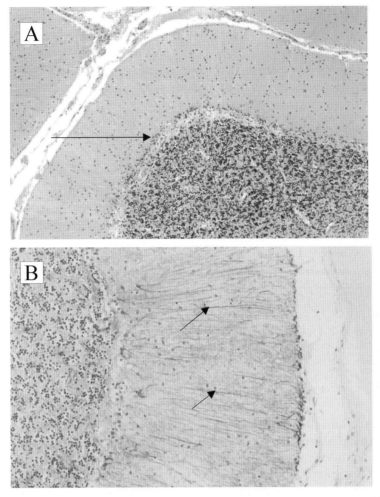

**Fig. 4** (A) Cerebellum showing evidence of previous hypoxic-ischaemic injury. Purkinje cells are depleted and instead a prominent row of glial nuclei are seen (arrow). The granule cell layer deep to this is preserved. (B) Immunohistochemistry to GFAP demonstrates glial processes (arrows) running in a linear fashion to the cerebellar cortical surface, characteristic of Bergmann gliosis.

Cellular events progress to necrosis and loss of neurons. Astrocytes respond with gliosis, which may be demonstrated using immunohistochemistry to glial fibrillary acidic protein (GFAP; Fig. 3). In the cerebellum, the loss of Purkinje cells is accompanied by Bergmann gliosis (Fig. 4A,B), a distinctive pattern of gliosis comprising increased numbers of reactive astrocytic nuclei along the Purkinje cell layer. Staining for GFAP highlights their processes which run radially to the cerebellar cortical surface. White matter in a brain subjected to a global hypoxic-ischaemic event will show oligodendroglial damage with myelin loss and gliosis at late time points.

Pathological assessment in a suspected case of ischaemic brain damage should involve a systematic assessment of vulnerable areas (Table 1). Macroscopic abnormalities may be subtle and the brain should be cut after fixation. Permission to retain the brain may be difficult to obtain, but it should

**Table 1** Assessment of hypoxic-ischaemic brain damage

- Obtain as full a clinical history as possible, including post-event survival interval
- The autopsy should include a full assessment of the cardiovascular system (see *Guidelines to the Stroke Autopsy*; <www.bns.org> BNS guidelines for good practice)
- Ideally cut the brain post-fixation
- Macroscopic assessment of the brain – carefully examine:
  * Cerebral arteries – multiple transverse cuts to document atheroma
  * Examine the entire cortical ribbon for areas of discolouration/laminar necrosis
  * Hippocampi
  * Arterial boundary zones
- Microscopic assessment – multiple vulnerable areas should be sampled including:
  * Areas of macroscopic abnormality
  * Hippocampi – both sides
  * Cortex – several blocks including boundary zones
  * Cerebellar cortex
  * Striatum
- Immunohistochemistry to GFAP helps in the assessment of gliosis
- CD68, a non-specific marker of microglial activation, can be helpful in characterising the extent of brain injury
- Examination of a single block of hippocampus is not an adequate assessment

be stressed that the examination may be impaired if the brain is cut in the fresh state. In addition to the sampling of macroscopically abnormal areas, blocks should be taken from areas known to be vulnerable to ischaemic brain damage including hippocampus, cerebellum, cerebral cortex (particularly from watershed areas), basal ganglia and central white matter.

## PATHWAYS TO CELL DEATH

Although there is some debate about the relative roles of apoptosis and necrosis in hypoxic-ischaemic injury, the predominant mode of neuronal death appears to be necrotic. Ischaemia leads to a fall in $PO_2$ with ensuing failure of membrane ATPases and membrane depolarisation. Associated efflux of glutamate into the extracellular space results in activation of the NMDA glutamate receptor, calcium influx into cells and resulting enzyme activation and generation of reactive oxygen species.[1,13] The concept of glutamate induced excitotoxicity would explain many aspects of ischaemic neuronal death, and the distribution of the NMDA receptors accounts for some aspects of the selective vulnerability of certain neuronal groups.[14] DNA damage also occurs in hypoxic-ischaemic injury due to oxidative damage. One consequence of this is the activation of the enzyme poly(ADP-ribose) polymerase (PARP) in response to single and double stranded DNA breaks. This enzyme results in the build-up of poly(ADP-ribose) groups on a variety of proteins, including histones. Cellular $NAD^+$ is consumed in this reaction and its depletion leads to impaired ATP synthesis which may contribute to the induction of cellular necrosis because of critical energy depletion.[15] In apoptosis, this process is prevented because PARP is cleaved by caspases. PARP and poly(ADP-ribose) groups are up-regulated in the post-ischaemic brain, suggesting a role for this process in hypoxic-ischaemic neuronal death.[13]

There is evidence that some cells also die by apoptosis,[16,17] and apoptosis has been suggested as a mechanism for delayed neuronal death. There is evidence of activation of apoptosis pathways, including caspase 3 in these cells. However, the morphology is generally not typical of apoptosis and DNA damage appears to be a late event so that some, but not all, of the features of apoptosis are present.[14,18,19] The assessment of cell death is compounded by the difficulty in identifying apoptosis, particularly in autopsy brain. The TUNEL method has been used extensively to identify apoptosis in tissue sections, but a positive reaction may also be seen in necrosis[20] and where endogenous endonucleases are activated.[18] Whilst identifying cells with DNA damage, the TUNEL technique needs to be interpreted critically and in the light of other techniques, in particular morphology and the expression of apoptosis regulatory molecules such as caspase 3.

The issue is further complicated because detailed morphological studies of neuronal death in a variety of CNS disorders suggest that a simple binary division of cell death into apoptotic or necrotic may be too simplistic. Whether apoptosis or necrosis is the outcome of a given cell stress may depend on the energy level of the cell.[21] The pathway of neuronal death in hypoxic-ischaemic injury might vary according to the severity of the insult. Morphological studies have suggested that neuronal death shows a continuum between apoptosis and necrosis.[19] An alternative suggestion is that there are a number of forms of cell death which have characteristics distinct from apoptosis or necrosis. This is supported by varying morphologies of neuronal death in a number of CNS disorders to which exotic names, such as aposklesis, abortosis and paraptosis, have been applied.[22]

How these variations apply to hypoxic-ischaemic neuronal death is currently uncertain but in ischaemia, as in other states in which neuronal death occurs, a classical dichotomy between apoptosis and necrosis seems inadequate to describe all of the cell death phenotypes observed. Further work is required to elucidate molecular and morphological pathways to death in the post-mitotic cell. Nevertheless, regulatory pathways do appear to operate. Even in the more common and clear-cut necrotic neuronal death, the role of molecules such as PARP suggests that there may be some degree of regulation and, therefore, a possibility of therapeutic intervention.

## THE EFFECTS OF DEVELOPMENT

The effects of hypoxic-ischaemic injury on the immature brain differ from those in the adult state. A detailed consideration of perinatal hypoxic-ischaemic brain damage is available in standard texts.[23] It is worth noting here that regions of greatest susceptibility are different from those in the adult. In perinatal global hypoxic-ischaemic injury, areas such as the pons, subiculum (combined in ponto-subicular necrosis), thalamus and brainstem are particularly susceptible. Often these forms of grey matter injury co-exist with germinal matrix haemorrhages and periventricular leukomalacia. The morphology of cell death also varies with developmental age in man and experimental systems; immature neurons are more likely to die by apoptosis.[19,24]

## THE NON-PERFUSED BRAIN – NOT TO BE CONFUSED WITH TRANSIENT GLOBAL HYPOXIC-ISCHAEMIC INJURY

The 'non-perfused brain' is a state that occurs after a global ischaemic event when there is no restoration of brain perfusion. The intracerebral pressure reaches a level such that cerebral perfusion is effectively zero. In some cases of raised intracranial pressure, vertebrobasilar flow is better maintained than carotid flow so that some brainstem functions may be preserved. Patients may be maintained on a ventilator for a variable time after such an event, hence the alternative names of respirator or ventilator brain for this condition. The pathological changes relate to non-perfusion rather than being specific to the effects of ventilation and non-perfused brain is the better term. Such a brain is swollen, dusky and grey; it may be softened and fragments of cerebellar cortex may be found in the subarachnoid space. The brain fixes poorly and often remains somewhat pink centrally. In contrast to transient global hypoxic-ischaemic injury with reperfusion, acidophilic ischaemic neuronal change is not a conspicuous feature though a few such neurons may be found. This emphasises the role of active processes associated with reperfusion in the evolution of morphological changes classically associated with ischaemia. Blood vessels appear dilated and red blood cells pale. In general, the brain shows no inflammatory response to these changes.[8,25]

## CELLULAR RESPONSES TO HYPOXIA

The ability of tissues to maintain oxygen homeostasis is essential for the survival of all cells which need to balance the production of ATP via oxidative phosphorylation against the risk of producing reactive oxygen species which are capable of damaging cellular DNA, lipids and proteins. It is now known that nearly all nucleated human cells are capable of sensing oxygen concentration and responding to hypoxic conditions. As in other physiological systems, adaptation to acute changes in oxygen concentration occurs via alterations (*e.g.* phosphorylation) of existing proteins, whereas adaptation to chronic changes in oxygenation result from alterations of gene expression. The understanding of these intracellular oxygen-sensing mechanisms at the molecular level is still in its infancy. Hypoxia and the cellular response to it are emerging as important contributors to a wide range of disorders. This section will focus on the role of two molecules, neuroglobin and hypoxia-inducible factor, that are emerging as important mediators of the cellular response to hypoxia in the brain and may be important in hypoxic-ischaemic injury and other cerebral diseases.

### NEUROGLOBIN

Cerebral tissue does not appear to have a mechanism, such as myoglobin, for the storage of oxygen. Recently, a novel globin, neuroglobin, has been found in brain. The role of this oxygen-binding protein is uncertain, but it may function to increase oxygen availability to neurons and its distribution is said to correlate anatomically with areas of selective vulnerability to hypoxia.[26,27] Hypoxia *in vitro* and cerebral ischaemia *in vivo* result in increased expression of neuroglobin in neurons: increased neuroglobin expression has a protective effect on neurons exposed to hypoxia. Both the induction of neuroglobin and its neuroprotective effects appear to be specific for hypoxia as the inducing insult.[28] Modulation of neuroglobin expression is, therefore, a potential therapeutic target for hypoxic-ischaemic brain injury and perhaps also for neurodegenerative diseases.

## HYPOXIA-INDUCIBLE FACTORS

A range of genes may be activated under hypoxic conditions. Many of these hypoxia-inducible genes appear to share a common method of regulation via activation of a transcription factors called the hypoxia-inducible factors (HIFs).[29] There are now several molecules in this family; most attention has focused on HIF-1α. HIFs activate the transcription of genes to form protein products which increase oxygen delivery (by stimulation of erythropoiesis and angiogenesis) or mediate metabolic adaptation to function under conditions of reduced oxygen availability (by stimulation of glycolytic enzymes, *etc.*). Experimental evidence suggests that under certain conditions HIF-regulated gene products (*e.g.* NIP3) may also mediate hypoxia-induced apoptosis. This protein, therefore, plays a pivotal role in the response to hypoxia.

### What are HIFs?

HIF-1 is a heterodimeric nuclear protein complex composed of HIF-1α and HIF-1β (also known as the aryl hydrocarbon nuclear translocator) subunits. Both subunits contain a basic helix-loop-helix PAS (bHLH/PAS) structure.[30] HIF-1β is constitutively expressed but the mRNA expression of HIF-1α, the half-life of its protein, and transactivation domain function are all regulated by cellular oxygen concentrations. HIF-1α is a prototype of this family of proteins and is specific to the HIF-1 heterodimer. An alternative dimerization partner for HIF-1β, which also activates genes via HIF-DNA recognition sites, has been variably named HIF-2α, HIF-1α-like factor, endothelial PAS domain protein 1 (EPAS-1), and mouse HIF-related factor.[31,32] HIF-1 binds to a specific consensus sequence in hypoxia-responsive enhancers/promoters of many target genes, where it interacts with other transcription factors bound at adjacent sites.

### Sites of normal expression

Both HIF-1α and HIF-2α mRNA have been shown to be expressed in many human cell lines.[32] *In situ* studies have shown that HIF-1α RNA is prevalent in all human tissues except in peripheral blood leukocytes and HIF-2α RNA is highly expressed in vascular tissue such as lung, heart, placenta and kidney.[31] Recent reports of immunostaining with a polyclonal antibody to HIF-1α in frozen tissue and monoclonal antibodies to HIF-1α and HIF-2α epitopes that survive formalin fixation and paraffin embedding have permitted extension of the study of expression and distribution of this protein family.[31,33] Most work on HIF-1α expression in brain tissue has been in the context of rats exposed to acute ischaemia. HIF-1α mRNA is present throughout the rat cortex and deep grey matter. The white matter in the corpus callosum and the internal capsule show very low expression[34] but the degree of its constitutive expression in deep subcortical white matter is unknown.

## The response to hypoxia

The expression of HIF-1 and HIF-1 transcriptional activity are precisely controlled by cellular oxygen concentrations. HIF-1β is constitutively expressed but HIF-1α is expressed at only low levels under normoxic conditions. With decreasing cellular oxygen concentrations, HIF-1 activity increases exponentially.[29] The exact molecular mechanisms by which changes in oxygen concentration lead to alterations in the activity of HIF-1 are poorly understood, but recent reports implicate a redox signal.[35] In non-hypoxic cells, the HIF-1α and HIF-2α proteins are ubiquitinated and undergo proteosomal degradation leading to inactivation. During hypoxia there is rapid intranuclear accumulation of HIF-1α[30] and HIF-2α.[31] They dimerize with HIF-1β, which makes them more resistant to proteolytic digestion, and bind to core DNA sequences of their target genes. They are rapidly degraded upon subsequent re-oxygenation. Therefore, HIF-1α and HIF-2α activities are regulated by the level of protein stability and not by mRNA levels.[32] Recently, groups of proteins capable of acting as co-repressors of the HIF-1 transactivation domain (*e.g.* VHL, FIH-1) have been identified.[36] Target genes activated by HIF-1 proteins include those controlling glucose/energy metabolism, cell viability, erythropoiesis, iron metabolism, vascular development and remodelling and others such as p53.[29] HIF-2α has an additional role in the regulation of VEGF receptor 2 (Fig. 5).[37]

Hypoxia is a major signal for inducing angiogenesis. The HIF family (HIF-1α and HIF-2α) plays an important role in modulating this process through the

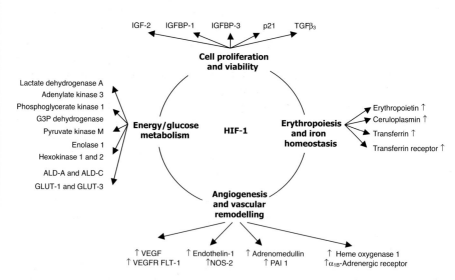

**Fig. 5** Gene expression induced by HIF activation. ALD-A and ALD–C, aldolase A and aldolase C; G3P, glyceraldehyde-3-phosphate; GLUT-1 and GLUT-3, glucose transporter 1 and 3; IGF-2, insulin-like growth factor 2; IGFBP-1 and IGFBP-3, insulin-like growth factor binding protein-1 and –3; PAI-1, plasminogen activator inhibitor; NOS-2, nitric oxide synthase 2; TGFβ₃, transforming growth factor β₃; VEGF, vascular endothelial growth factor; VEGFR FLT-1, vascular endothelial growth factor receptor FLT-1.

gene transcription of VEGF and VEGFR-1 and the protein expression of VEGFR-2. The expression of VEGF receptors indicates that the endothelium is maximally receptive to VEGF stimulation. It is thought that HIF-1 may co-ordinate VEGF signalling at multiple levels, similar to its regulation of many glucose transporters and glycolytic enzymes to provide metabolic adaptation. Recently, a role for VEGF in inducing interleukin 8 (IL-8) expression in human brain microvascular endothelial cells has been demonstrated which may be a possible mechanism for microglial activation in hypoxia.[38]

## CELLULAR RESPONSES TO HYPOXIA IN CNS DISORDERS

### Ischaemic and neurodegenerative diseases

Hypoxia is an important component of various forms of ischaemic brain damage, and there is evidence for a role for HIF in cerebral ischaemic states. The viable tissue around infarcts caused by permanent middle cerebral artery occlusion in adult rats shows increased expression of HIF-1$\alpha$ mRNA with a temporal and spatial correlation with the expression of mRNA of its target genes (GLUT-1, ALD-A, enolase-1, lactate dehydrogenase-A and other glycolytic enzymes).[34] HIF-1$\alpha$ and VEGF expression co-localise in the penumbra of an infarct preceding neovascularisation.[37]

These findings imply a role in the pathogenesis of acute ischaemic brain damage, especially in relation to repair and adaptation. In addition, there is evidence for a role for hypoxic response mechanisms in chronic vascular insufficiency. Deletion of the hypoxia-response element of the VEGF gene in the mouse has been shown to reduce hypoxia-induced VEGF expression in the spinal cord and causes an adult onset progressive motor neuron degeneration.[39] These mice have vascular perfusion deficits suggesting that chronic vascular insufficiency and impaired hypoxia-response mechanisms contribute to a neurodegenerative phenotype. Alternatively, VEGF may act as a neurotrophin by as yet undetermined signal pathways. These findings may well be relevant to human motor neuron diseases given the impairment of vascular perfusion with age and vulnerability of motor neurons to free radicals generated by hypoxia and ischaemia.

These links between vascular insufficiency and neurodegenerative disease suggest that hypoxia response mechanisms may also be involved in dementia states. Alzheimer's disease is the most common cause of dementia. It has been considered to be a purely neurodegenerative condition and since its first description more than 90 years ago, optimal patient management has been at best symptomatic. Over recent years, evidence has accumulated to suggest that Alzheimer's disease has a vascular component. The suggestion that non-genetic Alzheimer's disease is initiated by hypo-metabolism and ischaemia that precede the degenerative process has been fully reviewed elsewhere.[40] The hippocampus is vulnerable in Alzheimer's disease and in hypoxic-ischaemic injury. Levels of neuroglobin vary in different brain regions and are lower in the hippocampus.[26] It has recently been suggested that lower levels of this protein contribute to ischaemic susceptibility in this area, and that a reduced oxygen availability might be a contributing factor in Alzheimer's type pathology.[27] Such potential cellular mechanisms are intriguing, but currently remain speculative. A relation between vascular disease and Alzheimer's disease is also powerfully supported by epidemiological and clinical data on overlapping risk factors, similar cognitive symptoms, presence of similar vascular lesions, cerebral capillary degenerative patterns and results from therapeutic trials in both disorders.

Another pathological variable in dementing illnesses associated with brain hypoxia-ischaemia is the development of white matter lesions. Although their pathogenesis is not yet established, much of the evidence from clinical, pathological, and pathophysiological studies of human subjects favours a vascular mechanism.[41] Cellular components of white matter have been shown to be highly susceptible to ischaemia, and ICAM-1 and HIF up-regulation have also been demonstrated in white matter lesions.[42] They are frequent in Alzheimer's disease, a finding which further supports the concept that ischaemia/hypoxia plays a role in the development of this form of dementia.

## Hypoxia response mechanisms in neoplasia

Hypoxic areas develop in tumours with increasing tumour size and degree of malignancy. Hypoxia is a likely contributor to the increased levels of cell death by apoptosis and necrosis associated with malignant tumours. There is also evidence that hypoxia and the cellular adaptations to it have a role in a range of tumour-related processes, including angiogenesis and resistance to adjuvant therapies. It has been suggested that hypoxia may exert selective pressure within the tumour micro-environment contributing to tumour progression. Tumour cells developing a mutation, such as in the p53 gene, which abrogate hypoxia-induced apoptosis may compete with cells without the mutation and result in a more aggressive clone.[43,44]

Such mechanisms may well be important in gliomas. The most aggressive of the gliomas, the glioblastoma, is characterised by the presence of areas of necrosis and of endothelial proliferation. The tumour cells around such areas of necrosis are hypoxic and demonstrate expression of vascular endothelial growth factor which is important in angiogenesis in these tumours.[45] There is also increasing evidence for a role for HIF in glioma biology. In the diffusely infiltrating astrocytoma group (which, in increasing order of malignancy, includes the diffuse astrocytoma, anaplastic astrocytoma and glioblastoma multiforme), HIF-1α expression in gliomas increases with increasing aggressiveness and is, therefore, maximal in glioblastomas in which its expression is most prominent in cells adjacent to areas of necrosis suggesting that its induction is in response to hypoxia.[46,47] This is in contrast to the findings in haemangioblastoma in which diffuse expression of HIF-1α is thought to be related to mutation of the Von Hippel Lindau protein resulting in increased stabilisation of the protein.

Immunohistochemistry to HIF-1α appears useful as a means of identifying hypoxic areas in tumours and may also have some prognostic value. HIF-1α expression in oligodendrogliomas correlates with increased microvessel density and poorer prognosis.[48] Increased expression also appears to be a marker of more aggressive disease in non-CNS tumours including breast and cervical cancer. Through its ability to transactivate a range of genes (Fig. 5), expression of HIF may confer a selective advantage to a tumour. For example, it may promote angiogenesis via VEGF, extend cell survival via insulin-like growth factor, and affect metabolism through induced expression of glucose transporters.[29] There is also evidence for an interaction with p53. HIF-1α mediates the hypoxia-induced activation of p53, binding to the protein to stabilise it.[49] Loss of p53 activity, through mutation, reduces hypoxia-induced cell death,[43] but p53 also inhibits HIF activity by targeting HIF-1α for Mdm-2 mediated degradation. Loss of p53 amplifies hypoxia-induced levels of HIF with consequent increases in VEGF levels and angiogenesis.[50] Therefore, HIF activation may be brought into play via several mechanisms and contribute to tumour pathogenesis.

## ACKNOWLEDGEMENTS

Work in this laboratory is supported by the Medical Research Council, UK. Dr M.S. Fernando is supported by the Association of Commonwealth Universities.

---

### Points of best practice

- The effects of pure hypoxic states differ from hypoxic-ischaemic brain damage.

- Transient global hypoxia-ischaemia may produce widespread brain damage the distribution of which is affected by vascular territories and selective vulnerability of certain neuronal types.

- Neurons are more vulnerable than glia to acute hypoxic-ischaemic injury. Neurons within the CA1 region of the hippocampus, layers 3 and 5 of the cerebral cortex and the Purkinje cells of the cerebellum are particularly vulnerable.

- Widespread sampling is essential for the assessment of hypoxic-ischaemic brain damage.

- Most neurons die by necrosis after hypoxia-ischaemia, but some may die by apoptosis.

- Cells are able to respond to hypoxia by up-regulation of hypoxia inducible factor. This in turn transactivates genes affecting cell metabolism, survival and angiogenesis.

- Hypoxia and hypoxia inducible factor may play a role in the pathogenesis of a range of CNS disorders, including tumours and degenerative diseases of the ageing brain.

---

### References

1. Erecinska M, Silver IA. Tissue oxygen tension and brain sensitivity to hypoxia. *Respir Physiol* 2001; **128**: 263–276.
2. Auer RN, Sutherland GR. Hypoxia and related conditions. In: Graham DI, Lantos PL. (eds) *Greenfield's Neuropathology*, 7th edn, vol 1. London: Arnold, 2002; 233–280.
3. Gray FD, Horner JH. Survival following extreme hypoxia. *JAMA* 1970; **211**: 1815–1817.
4. Sadove MS, Yon MK, Hollinger PH, Johnston KS, Phillips FL. Severe prolonged cerebral hypoxic episode with complete recovery. *JAMA* 1961; **174**: 1102–1104.

5. Rie MA, Benad PG. Prolonged hypoxia in man without circulatory compromise fails to demonstrate cerebral pathology. *Neurology* 1980; **30**: 443.
6. Miyamoto O, Auer RN. Hypoxia, hyperoxia, ischaemia and brain necrosis. *Neurology* 2000; **54**: 362–371.
7. Pearigen P, Gwinn R, Simon RP. The effects *in vivo* of hypoxia on brain injury. *Brain Res* 1996; **725**: 184–191.
8. Garcia JH. Morphology of global cerebral ischaemia. *Crit Care Med* 1988; **16**: 979–987.
9. Brierley JB, Meldrum BS, Brown AW. The threshold and neuropathology of cerebral 'anoxic-ischaemic' cell change. *Arch Neurol* 1973; **29**: 367–373.
10. Evans TJ, Krausz T. Pathogenesis and pathology of shock. In: Anthony PP, MacSween RNM. (eds) *Recent Advances in Histopathology*, vol 16. Edinburgh: Churchill Livingstone, 1994; 21–47.
11. Brierley JB, Graham DI, Adams JH, Simpson JA. Neocortical death after cardiac arrest. *Lancet* 1971; **ii**: 560–565.
12. Petito CK, Feldman E, Pulsinelli WA, Plum F. Delayed hippocampal damage in humans following cardiorespiratory arrest. *Neurology* 1987; **37**: 1281–1286.
13. Love S. Oxidative stress in brain ischaemia. *Brain Pathol* 1999; **9**: 119–131.
14. Kirino T. Delayed neuronal death. *Neuropathology* 2000; **20 (Suppl.)**: 95–97.
15. D'Amours D, Desnoyers S, D'Silva I, Poirier GG. Poly(ADP-ribosyl)ation reactions in the regulation of nuclear functions. *Biochem J* 1999; **342**: 249–268.
16. Choi DW. Ischaemia-induced neuronal apoptosis. *Curr Opin Neurobiol* 1996; **6**: 667–672.
17. Yuan J, Yanker BA. Apoptosis in the nervous system. *Nature* 2000; **407**: 802–809.
18. Love S, Barber R, Wilcock GK. Neuronal death in brain infarcts in man. *Neuropathol Appl Neurobiol* 2000; **26**: 55–66.
19. Martin LJ, Al-Abdulla NA, Brambrink AM *et al.* Neurodegeneration in excitotoxicity, global cerebral ischaemia and target deprivation: a perspective on the contributions of apoptosis and necrosis. *Brain Res Bull* 1998; **46**: 281–309.
20. Grasl-Kraupp B, Ruttkay-Nedecky B, Koudelka H *et al. In situ* detection of fragmented DNA (TUNEL assay) fails to discriminate among apoptosis, necrosis, and autolytic cell death: a cautionary note. *Hepatology* 1995; **21**: 1465–1468.
21. Leist M, Single B, Castoldi AF, Kühnle S, Nicotera P. Intracellular adenosine triphosphate (ATP) concentration: a switch in the decision between apoptosis and necrosis. *J Exp Med* 1997; **185**: 1481–1486.
22. Graeber MB, Moran LR. Mechanisms of cell death in neurodegenerative diseases: fashion, fiction and facts. *Brain Pathol* 2002; **12**: 385–390.
23. Kinney HC, Armstrong DD. Perinatal neuropathology. In: Graham DI, Lantos PL. (eds) Greenfield's Neuropathology, 7th edn, vol 1. London: Arnold, 2002; 519–606.
24. Edwards AD, Mehmet H. Apoptosis in perinatal hypoxic-ischaemic cerebral damage. *Neuropathol Appl Neurobiol* 1996; **22**: 494–498.
25. Grunnet ML, Paulson G. Pathological changes in irreversible brain death. *Dis Nerv Syst* 1971; **32**: 690–694.
26. Burmester T, Welch B, Reinhardt S, Hankein T. A vertebrate globin expressed in the brain. *Nature* 2000; **407**: 520–523.
27. Moens L, Dewilde S. Globins in the brain. *Nature* 2000; **407**: 461–462.
28. Sun Y, Jin K, Mao XO, Zhu Y, Greenberg DA. Neuroglobin is up-regulated by and protects neurons from hypoxic-ischemic injury. *Proc Natl Acad Sci USA* 2001; **98**: 15306–15311.
29. Semenza GL. HIF-1 and tumor progression: pathophysiology and therapeutics. *Trends Mol Med* 2002; **8 (Suppl.)**: 62–67.
30. Wang GL, Jiang B-H, Rue EA, Semenza GL. Hypoxia-inducible factor 1 is a basic-helix-loop-helix-PAS heterodimer regulated by cellular $O_2$ tension. *Proc Natl Acad Sci USA* 1995; **92**: 5510–5514.
31. Talks KL, Turley H, Gatter KC *et al.* The expression and distribution of the hypoxia-inducible factors HIF-1 alpha and HIF-2 alpha in normal human tissues, cancers, and tumour associated macrophages. *Am J Pathol* 2000; **157**: 411–421.
32. Wiesener MS, Turley H, Allen WE *et al.* Induction of endothelial PAS domain protein-1 by hypoxia: characterisation and comparison with hypoxia-inducible factor-1 alpha. *Blood* 1998; **92**: 2260–2268.

33. Zhong H, De Marzo AM, Laughner E *et al*. Overexpression of hypoxia-inducible factor 1 alpha in common human cancers and their metastases. *Cancer Res* 1999; **59**: 5830–5935.

34. Bergeron M, Gidday JM, Yu AY *et al*. Role of hypoxia-inducible factor 1 in hypoxia induced tolerance in neonatal rat brain. *Ann Neurol* 2000; **48**: 285–296.

35. Chandel NS, Schumacker PT. Cellular oxygen sensing by mitochondria: old questions, new insight. *J Appl Physiol* 2000; **88**: 1880–1889.

36. Mahon PC, Hirota K, Semenza GL. FIH-1: a novel protein that interacts with HIF-1 alpha and VHL to mediate repression of HIF-1 transcriptional activity. *Genes Dev* 2002; **15**: 2675–2686.

37. Marti HJ, Bernaudin M, Bellail A *et al*. Hypoxia-induced vascular endothelial growth factor expression precedes neovascularisation after cerebral ischaemia. *Am J Pathol* 2000; **156**: 965–976.

38. Lee T-H, Avraham H, Lee SH, Avraham S. Vascular endothelial growth factor modulates neutrophil transendothelial migration via upregulation of interleukin-8 in human brain microvascular endothelial cells. *J Biol Chem* 2002; **277**: 10445–10451.

39. Oosthuyse B, Moons L, Storkebaum E *et al*. Deletion of the hypoxia-response element in the vascular endothelial growth factor promoter causes motor neuron degeneration. *Nat Genet* 2001; **28**: 131–138.

40. De la Torre JC. Alzheimer's disease as a vascular disorder: nosological evidence. *Stroke* 2002; **33**: 1152–1162.

41. Pantoni L, Garcia JH. Pathogenesis of leukoaraiosis. A review. *Stroke* 1997; **28**: 652–659.

42. Ince PG, Fernando MS. Evidence for an ischaemic origin of deep white matter lesions in the ageing brain. *Neuropathol Appl Neurobiol* 2002; **28**: 150–151.

43. Graeber TG, Osmanian C, Jacks M *et al*. Hypoxia-mediated selection of cells with diminished apoptotic potential in solid tumours. *Nature* 1996; **379**: 88–91.

44. Royds JA, Dower SK, Qwarnstrom EE, Lewis CE. Response of tumour cells to hypoxia: role of p53 and NF-κB. *J Clin Pathol Mol Pathol* 1998; **51**: 55–61.

45. Kleihues P, Burger PC, Collins VP *et al*. Glioblastoma. In: Kleihues P, Cavanee WK. (eds) *Tumours of the Nervous System*. Lyon: IARC, 2000; 29–39.

46. Sondergaard KL, Hilton DA, Penney M, Ollerenshaw M, Demaine AG. Expression of hypoxia-inducible factor 1α in tumours of patients with glioblastoma. *Neuropathol Appl Neurobiol* 2002; **28**: 210–217.

47. Zagzag D, Zhong H, Scalzitti JM *et al*. Expression of hypoxia-inducible factor 1α in brain tumors. *Cancer* 2000; **88**: 2606–2618.

48. Birner P, Gatterbauer B, Oberhuber G *et al*. Expression of hypoxia-inducible factor-1α in oligodendrogliomas. *Cancer* 2001; **92**: 165–171.

49. An WG, Kanekal M, Simon MC *et al*. Stabilisation of wild-type p53 by hypoxia-inducible factor 1α. *Nature* 1998; **392**: 405–408.

50. Ravi R, Mookerjee B, Bhujwalla ZM *et al*. Regulation of tumour angiogenesis by p53-induced degradation by hypoxia-inducible factor 1α. *Genes Dev* 2000; **14**: 34–44.

*Bridget S. Wilkins   David Clark*

10

# Recent advances in bone marrow pathology

Bone marrow trephine biopsy has become such an established part of the haematological diagnostic repertoire that it is perhaps surprising to recall that the first needles designed specifically for this purpose (Islam and Jamshedi) became widely used only from the mid 1970s. It is now relatively uncommon for bone marrow aspiration to be done without a trephine biopsy and the complementary value of these two investigations is unchallenged. In recent years, advances in the field of bone marrow pathology have included developments in biopsy needle design, modifications to specimen processing, advances in immunohistochemistry and molecular diagnostic techniques, and new insights into histological features of bone marrow physiology and pathology. The evolution of lymphoma classification systems in recent years has also been of importance for bone marrow pathology. In particular, the World Health Organization's (WHO) classification introduced at the end of 1999 is the first to encompass myeloproliferative as well as lympho-proliferative disorders in a single system.[1] Crucially, the WHO approach is multidisciplinary and its aim is to define clinicopathologically relevant disease entities. It is intended to be flexible, particularly with regard to incorporating the increasing contribution of genetic data to diagnostic and prognostic evaluation of haematological neoplasia. For the first time in lymphoma classification, the contribution that the histological appearances of infiltrates in bone marrow can make to diagnosis receives mention. However, the usefulness of such information from trephine histology is still insufficiently recognised.

**Dr Bridget S. Wilkins** DM PhD FRCPath
Consultant Histopathologist, Pathology Department, Royal Victoria Infirmary, Queen Victoria Road, Newcastle upon Tyne NE1 4LP, UK (for correspondence)

**Dr David Clark** MD MRCP FRCPath
Consultant Histopathologist,Pathology Department, Grantham and Kesteven District Hospital, Manthorpe Road, Grantham NG31 8DG, UK

## TECHNICAL ADVANCES

### NEEDLES

The original Islam and Jamshedi trephine biopsy needles were robust, re-usable needle-and-trocar units that were sterilised by autoclaving and could be re-sharpened when necessary. Disposable needles were initially developed to ensure adequate sharpness for every trephine biopsy, as older re-usable units tended to blunt ever more easily with long-term use. The relatively high cost of disposable needles limited their uptake in the UK until concerns about possible transmission of prion proteins via re-used needles effectively mandated their use. In recent years, further advances in needle technology have largely been aimed at improving capture and retrieval of the tissue core. Modern needle designs incorporate additional cutting devices or spring traps. These minimise the potentially damaging mechanical effort required to break off the inner end of the core and ensure that the core is withdrawn cleanly within the hollow needle. Powered myelotomy drills,[2] requiring general anaesthesia and open biopsy procedures, have not become widely accepted in haematological practice. Bone marrow trephine biopsy, therefore, remains largely a manual skill of the haematologist. The expertise of the operator and the size of needle used (the larger the better for specimen integrity) remain the most important determinants of a successful biopsy.

### PROCESSING

Most bone marrow trephine biopsies are fixed in formaldehyde-based solutions though Bouin's is favoured in a few centres for possible minor benefits in cytological preservation. In the 1980s, enthusiasm for plastic embedding without decalcification reached a high point but has since waned. This has mostly been a reflection of the increased requirement for immunohistochemistry on bone marrow sections. The relatively high cost of plastic embedding and the necessity to maintain technical skills not otherwise needed in most histopathology laboratories has also contributed. Immunohistochemical techniques are successful on plastic sections but non-standard pretreatments and antibody dilutions are required. This makes incorporation into the routine immuno-histochemical work of histopathology laboratories difficult, particularly with increased automation of immunostaining.

Consequently, most laboratories decalcify bone marrow trephine biopsies after formalin fixation using organic acids or chelating agents. The former have been favoured traditionally because they work quicker than chelation. New requirements for preservation of nucleic acids in trephine biopsy specimens, for molecular genetic techniques such as PCR and ISH, are changing practice in this aspect of processing. Use of the chelating agent EDTA has been shown to permit retrieval of high molecular weight DNA (600 bp) from archival, routinely processed bone marrow cores.[3] The quality of DNA from acid-decalcified cores was considerably less with only rare retrieval of fragments more than 200 bp in length.[4]

Use of chelating agents for trephine biopsy decalcification causes no detri-mental effect on histological quality or the success of immunohistochemistry.

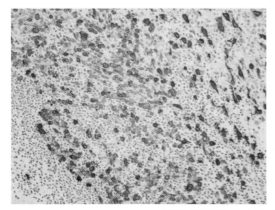

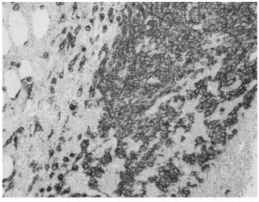

**Fig. 1** Neoplastic mast cells in indolent mastocytosis. Immuno-histochemical staining for (a) tryptase and (b) c-kit. Original magnification x20.

Preservation of a degree of enzyme activity in bone marrow cells with this technique, unlike with acid decalcification, has the added benefit of permitting successful use of Leder's stain (chloro-acetate esterase), an excellent method for demonstrating the distribution of granulopoietic cells in bone marrow sections.

Any reluctance to adopt a slower decalcifying method will surely be overcome in the next few years as microwave processing techniques are refined and become more widely used in histopathology laboratories. Potentially, microwave heating can be used to increase the speed of initial fixation, reduce decalcification time and provide rapid tissue processing through solvents into wax. Data are not yet available to indicate whether or not microwave processing impairs preservation of nucleic acid in tissue biopsies. It seems unlikely that it should, providing that initial tissue fixation is adequate.

## IMMUNOHISTOCHEMISTRY

As with other tissues, widespread adoption of wet-heat antigen retrieval methods has expanded the range of immunohistochemistry applicable to trephine biopsy sections. Much of the extended target range is by now familiar but recent additions include c-kit (CD117) and tartrate-resistant acid phosphatase (TRAP). Demonstration of c-kit expression is a useful addition to tryptase staining in confirming mast cell infiltration (Fig. 1). It may also prove helpful in characterising blast cells in myelodysplastic syndromes and acute myeloid leukaemias as it highlights haemopoietic precursor cells at a more immature stage than can be detected by CD34 expression. Staining for TRAP offers specific confirmation of hairy cell leukaemia; previously, DBA44[5] was the best available paraffin wax-reactive antibody for this purpose. DBA44 is not entirely specific: some cases of other forms of small B-cell lymphoma may stain positively. Staining for TRAP with new antibody clones tends to give a degree of background positivity in haemopoietic tissue, so that subtle interstitial infiltration and minimal residual disease after treatment may be missed. A robust pan-B cell marker such as CD20 should always be used in addition to TRAP or the antigen detected by DBA44 in these contexts to quantify the extent of infiltration.

New uses for established antibodies are also being found. Staining for CD34 in the assessment of myelodysplastic and myeloproliferative conditions is described below. Use of CD42b or CD61 staining of megakaryocytes to assess their number, distribution, size and cytological detail is proving particularly helpful in differentiating normal or reactive haemopoiesis from that of myelodysplastic or chronic myeloproliferative states. In the context of suspected lymphoproliferative disease, demonstration of rough endoplasmic reticulum associated p63 antigen (antibody VS38c)[6] or CD138 is useful to highlight plasma cells in patients with monoclonal gammopathy of undetermined significance (MGUS). Immunostaining for kappa and lambda light chains is often difficult to interpret in trephine biopsies because of sensitivity of decalcified tissue to proteolytic antigen retrieval methods and the high content of plasma in marrow interstitium. A recent innovation has been the development of immunofluorescent methods suitable for decalcified, routinely processed trephine sections.[7] This permits dual staining of kappa and lambda chains in a section with different fluorochromes so that the ratio of the two can be determined directly. As with streptavidin-biotin based immuno-histochemical methods, however, sensitivity of this immunofluorescent method is insufficient to detect surface immunoglobulin expressed on lymphoid cells other than plasma cells.

## MOLECULAR BIOLOGY

*In situ* hybridisation (ISH) for mRNA currently has only a limited role in diagnostic histopathology. One application is for the demonstration of kappa and lambda light chain expression by plasma cells in bone marrow. Commercially available kits permit easy detection of kappa and lambda mRNA, with high positive signal strength and no background staining (Fig. 2). This approach avoids the technical and interpretative difficulties inherent in the use of immunohistochemistry to demonstrate light chain proteins. Like immunohistochemistry, ISH is currently only sensitive enough to detect abundant molecules in plasma cell cytoplasm. It cannot reliably be used to demonstrate light chain restriction in non-plasma cell lymphoid proliferations. In the context of suspected bone marrow involvement by Hodgkin's disease or post-transplant lymphoproliferative disease, ISH kits to demonstrate Epstein-Barr virus early RNA species (EBV-EBER) can be used successfully to demonstrate EBV latency in neoplastic lymphoid cells.

The RNA ISH kits usually use chromogenic substrates for signal detection. Detection of DNA targets by ISH generally uses fluorescently labelled chromo-

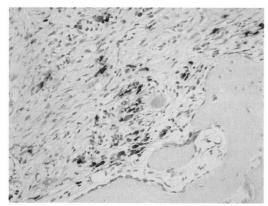

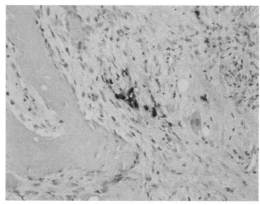

**Fig. 2** Polytypic, reactive plasma cells within osteosclerotic bone marrow. *In situ* hybridisation for (a) kappa and (b) lambda immunoglobulin light chain mRNA. Trephine biopsy was performed to investigate possible osteosclerotic myeloma but was found instead to show rare clusters of metastatic carcinoma cells. Original magnification x20.

some paints, centromeric probes or sequence-specific probes. These are all used in the diagnosis of haematological malignancies using aspirated blood or bone marrow cells. So far, their application to trephine biopsy sections has been limited by technical constraints but methods have been developed to overcome these. Several research groups have now reported successful demonstration of chromosomal abnormalities in bone marrow cells in trephine sections.[8,9] Numerical abnormalities (gain or absence of a chromosome paint or centromeric probe signal) and translocations (localisation of dual or multiple signals from differently labelled probes in the same nuclei) have been demonstrated. The major technical constraint in applying FISH in trephines, as for any histological sections, is the need to take into account the fact that only a slice of each nucleus is represented. Whole nuclei can be extracted from thick sections and prepared as cytospin films, as for other histological specimens, but this obviously entails loss of tissue architecture. For haematological malignancies, unless the disease is associated with severe hypoplasia or marrow fibrosis, there will usually be an aspirated cell preparation to be used in preference, as long as such use is anticipated when samples are collected.

PCR can be performed with template DNA extracted from trephine biopsy sections as mentioned above. Non-standard fixatives have proved helpful in preserving DNA in some studies but generally have drawbacks such as impaired preservation of cytological detail or restriction of the range of effective immunohistochemistry. Standard formalin fixation followed by

EDTA decalcification offers a good alternative with excellent morphological and antigenic preservation. The only drawback is that decalcification takes longer than with formic or acetic acid. Applications of DNA PCR are mainly of interest in the context of lymphoma diagnosis or residual disease detection (clonality studies, *BCL-1* and *BCL-2* re-arrangement analyses). The balanced translocations associated with many forms of myeloid neoplasia involve chromosomal breakpoints distributed over wide areas which makes PCR primer design a great problem. Using fresh blood or bone marrow cells, RT-PCR has been adopted as an alternative approach for targets such as *BCR-ABL*, *PML-RARA* and *AML1-ETO*. Methods have been developed in recent years to permit extraction of sufficiently high quality mRNA from formalin-fixed tissues for reverse transcription followed by PCR.[10] As yet, these methods have not been applied successfully to routinely processed, decalcified bone marrow specimens but it is probably only a matter of time and experimentation before this technical challenge is overcome.

## THE BONE MARROW BIOPSY IN MYELOID NEOPLASIA – IMPLICATIONS OF THE WHO CLASSIFICATION

Most pathologists in the UK have readily become familiar with the WHO classification system for lymphoid neoplasia,[1] in large part because it builds upon the success of the REAL classification[11] which had already gained widespread international acceptance. However, there is less familiarity and less widespread acceptance of the WHO classification system for the other haemopoietic neoplasms (acute myeloid leukaemias, myelodysplasias and chronic myeloproliferative diseases) published in the same monograph.[1] The WHO panel adopted the same approach for myeloid neoplasms that had been taken with lymphoid neoplasms. Clinical, haematological, histopathological, immunophenotypic and molecular genetic features are used to define entities with distinct biological features and behaviour. The new WHO classification incorporates aspects of previous systems, such as the French-American-British (FAB)[12,13] and the morphological, immunological, cytogenetic, molecular genetic (MIC-M)[14,15] classifications of myeloid proliferations. These have been established in use by haematologists and have stood the test of time. However, many histopathologists in the UK are unfamiliar with the detail of previous classification systems for these diseases, in part because histopathological features did not contribute to the formal diagnostic criteria for most of these conditions. Nonetheless, most haematologists and haematopathologists recognise that there are many ways in which the bone marrow biopsy is of great diagnostic value in myeloid neoplasia. Trephine biopsy histology provides additional information that cannot be derived from aspirated bone marrow, such as disturbances of normal haemopoietic micro-architecture and the presence of bone marrow fibrosis. This deficiency has been addressed by the WHO classification and histopathological features have now been incorporated into formal diagnostic criteria for many neoplastic myeloid diseases.

The WHO classifies myeloid haemopoietic neoplasms into four broad groups – chronic myeloproliferative diseases, myeloproliferative/myelodysplastic diseases, myelodysplastic syndromes, and acute myeloid leukaemias. The following

**Table 1** WHO classification of chronic myeloproliferative diseases

| |
|---|
| Chronic myelogenous leukaemia (Philadelphia chromosome, t9;22)(q34;q11), BCR/ABL positive) |
| Chronic neutrophilic leukaemia |
| Chronic eosinophilic leukaemia (and the hypereosinophilic syndrome) |
| Polycythaemia vera |
| Chronic idiopathic myelofibrosis (with extramedullary haemopoiesis) |
| Essential thrombocythaemia |
| Chronic myeloproliferative disease, unclassifiable |

discussion will highlight areas in which the WHO monograph identifies bone marrow histological findings as being of diagnostic importance or providing prognostic information.

## CHRONIC MYELOPROLIFERATIVE DISEASES

The chronic myeloproliferative diseases (Table 1) are clonal disorders derived from haemopoietic stem cells in which there is proliferation of haemopoietic precursors with maturation and overproduction of cells from one or more lineage.[16,17]

Chronic myeloid leukaemia is defined by the presence of the Philadelphia chromosome, t(9;22) and/or the *BCR-ABL* fusion gene. The disease is characterised by an initial chronic phase (CML-CP) in which there is leukocytosis with immature granulocytic precursors in the peripheral blood. The disease transforms into a blast phase (CML-BP) which resembles an acute leukaemia. CML-BP is often preceded by an accelerated phase (CML-AP). The finding of severe megakaryocytic proliferation, with large sheets or clusters of megakaryocytes, associated with dense reticulin or collagen deposition in bone marrow trephine sections is suggestive of progression to CML-AP.[18] CML-BP may be diagnosed when there are large foci or clusters of blast cells even if the other histological appearances are typical of CML-CP. Care should be taken not to confuse promyelocytes (which are often present in increased numbers in paratrabecular and peri-arteriolar areas in CML-CP) with blast cells. Immunohistochemical staining for CD34 is often helpful in identifying blast cells.[19]

Chronic neutrophilic leukaemia and chronic eosinophilic leukaemia are rare conditions characterised by leukocytosis with a predominance of neutrophils and eosinophils, respectively. The principal role of bone marrow trephine histology in these contexts is to exclude other conditions that result in leukocytosis, such as early stage chronic idiopathic myelofibrosis.

Polycythaemia vera (PV) is characterised by excessive production of red blood cells unresponsive to the normal negative feedback mechanisms that regulate their production. Diagnosis of PV requires the demonstration of a raised red cell mass in the absence of an identifiable cause of reactive, secondary erythrocytosis in combination with at least one other major (A) or two minor (B) diagnostic criteria.[20] Abnormal bone marrow histology is one of the B criteria. The bone marrow is usually hypercellular with erythroid

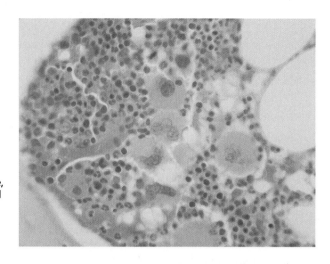

**Fig. 3** Loosely clustered megakaryocytes in PV showing variation in size, nuclear morphology and nucleus:cytoplasm ratio. H&E-stained section; original magnification x40.

hyperplasia and normoblastic erythropoiesis. There is usually megakaryocytic proliferation with clustering of megakaryocytes around sinusoids. The megakaryocytes typically show nuclear pleomorphism (Fig. 3) with large hyperlobated and small hypolobated forms.[20,21] There is an increase in stromal reticulin in about 30% of cases. Some patients progress to a 'spent' phase of disease in which anaemia supervenes and bone marrow histology shows severe collagen fibrosis. The fibrosis may be indistinguishable from that of chronic idiopathic myelofibrosis if the history of preceding PV is not known.

Chronic idiopathic myelofibrosis (CIMF) is another clonal haemopoietic stem cell disorder in which there is predominant megakaryocytic and granulocytic proliferation with reactive bone marrow fibrosis. About 20–30% of patients present in a pre-fibrotic stage sometimes referred to as 'cellular phase' CIMF.[22,23] Bone marrow trephine sections in this cellular phase show hypercellular haemopoiesis with granulocytic and megakaryocytic hyperplasia. The megakaryocytes vary in size and shape with a predominance of large cells showing abnormal nuclear lobation and hyperchromasia.[24] Typically, clusters of megakaryocytes are seen in paratrabecular and perisinusoidal positions. In the cellular phase of CIMF there is little increase in reticulin. Most patients present in the fibrotic phase of the disease, which is characterised by severe bone marrow fibrosis, decreased haemopoietic cellularity, dilated stromal sinusoids and intrasinusoidal haemopoiesis. Megakaryocytes are increased in number, with clustering of cells and severe nuclear atypia. Appositional new bone formation around trabeculae is common, causing osteosclerosis.

Essential thrombocythaemia (ET) is a myeloproliferative disease in which there is overproduction of platelets. Diagnosis requires two positive diagnostic criteria – a sustained elevation of the platelet count (> 600 x $10^9$/l) and abnormal bone marrow histology. The latter is characterised by normal or only moderately hypercellular haemopoiesis with increased numbers of megakaryocytes. Megakaryocytes in ET are typically large with voluminous cytoplasm and enlarged, hyperlobated nuclei having well-separated nuclear lobes (Fig. 4).[25,26] Loose clusters of megakaryocytes are usually present.

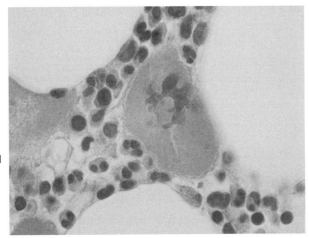

**Fig. 4** Large megakaryo-cyte in ET showing voluminous cytoplasm and a hyperlobated nucleus with well separated nuclear lobes ('staghorn nucleus'). H&E-stained section; original magnification x100.

Reticulin fibrosis is minimal or absent, an important feature in distinguishing ET from those cases of CIMF presenting with a raised platelet count. Diagnosis also requires the exclusion of other specific myeloproliferative diseases in which an elevated platelet count may be found (particularly CML and PV) and conditions associated with reactive thrombocytosis. Recently, demonstration of abnormal c-mpl expression by megakaryocytes in ET has been suggested as a potential new diagnostic tool.[27] c-mpl is the thrombopoietin receptor expressed by megakaryocytes and their precursor cells.

Cases in which there are clinical, haematological and histological features of a myeloproliferative disease but which fail to fulfil diagnostic criteria of any of the specific myeloproliferative disorders described above are designated chronic myeloproliferative disease unclassifiable (MPD-U).[28] Two broad groups of cases are recognised on the basis of bone marrow histology. The first consists of early stage cases which probably represent CIMF, ET and PV in which diagnostic features have not fully emerged. It is not clear from the criteria described in the WHO monograph how this pattern of MPD-U can be distinguished from cellular phase CIMF. The second group of cases is characterised by extensive myelofibrosis resembling fibrotic phase CIMF or post-PV myelofibrosis. In practice, most patients presenting with this pattern of bone marrow histology will probably meet the diagnostic criteria for CIMF.

## MYELOPROLIFERATIVE/MYELODYSPLASTIC DISEASES

These disorders, as the name implies, have both dysplastic and proliferative features.[29] Four entities are recognised, all of which present clinically as chronic leukaemias (Table 2). The histological features seen in bone marrow trephine sections are not specific. In all MPD/MDS there is granulocytic hyperplasia accompanied by variable dysplasia of erythroid cells and megakaryocytes. Some cases have haematological and clinical features of one of the categories of myelodysplasia and also have myeloproliferative features (*e.g.* a raised platelet count). They lack defining cytogenetic or molecular genetic features of a specific MPD or MDS (*e.g.* t(9;22), *BCR-ABL* re-arrangement or del 5q). The term MPD/MDS unclassifiable (MPD/MDS-U) is

**Table 2** WHO classification of myelodysplastic/myeloproliferative diseases

Chronic myelomonocytic leukaemia

Atypical chronic myeloid leukaemia

Juvenile myelomonocytic leukaemia

Myelodysplastic/myeloproliferative disease, unclassifiable

used to designate such cases.

## MYELODYSPLASIA

The myelodysplastic syndromes are a group of clonal haemopoietic stem cell disorders in which there is ineffective haemopoiesis leading to cytopenias affecting one or more of the haemopoietic cell lineages (Table 3).[16,30]. Many cases undergo clonal evolution and transform into acute myeloid leukaemia. The classification of myelodysplasia is dependent on the peripheral blood and bone marrow aspirate findings. A bone marrow biopsy provides useful additional evidence of dysplasia of haemopoietic cells and is particularly helpful in cases with bone marrow fibrosis or severe hypoplasia of the marrow.

In low-grade myelodysplasia (refractory anaemia and refractory anaemia with ring sideroblasts)[30] the bone marrow usually shows varying degrees of hyperplasia with dyserythopoiesis. The granulocytic precursors and megakaryocytes do not usually have morphological evidence of dysplasia. These findings are relatively non-specific and can be seen in a variety of non-neoplastic conditions such as vitamin $B_{12}$ and folate deficiency or as a result of chemotherapeutic agents.[15] It is crucially important to interpret the morphological features in the light of all available clinical and haematological information.

In the higher grade myelodysplasias (refractory cytopenia with multilineage dysplasia and refractory anaemia with excess of blasts)[30] there is usually evidence of megakaryocytic dysplasia: the megakaryocytes are typically small with a hypolobated nucleus and high nucleus:cytoplasm ratio. Less commonly, these cells are of normal size with multiple small separate nuclei. Megakaryocytes may also be seen in abnormal paratrabecular sites. Granulocytic dysplasia is not usually detectable in histological sections from bone marrow trephine cores unless there is abnormal localisation of immature precursors (ALIP). ALIP is defined as the

**Table 3** The WHO classification of myelodysplastic syndromes

Refractory anaemia

Refractory anaemia with ringed sideroblasts

Refractory cytopenia with multilineage dysplasia

Refractory anaemia with excess blasts

Myelodysplastic syndrome, unclassifiable

Myelodysplastic syndrome associated with isolated del(5q) chromosomal abnormality presence of three or more clusters containing 5–8 myeloblasts or promyelocytes away from their normal positions in paratrabecular and peri-arteriolar regions.[30] Refractory anaemia with excess of blasts is characterised histologically by increased numbers of myeloblasts. Immunohistochemical staining for CD34 is helpful in demonstrating blast cells in bone marrow trephine biopsy sections[31] and in highlighting ALIP. This is particularly valuable in the differentiation of hypoplastic myelodysplasia in which CD34-positive cells are increased in number and in aplastic anaemia in which CD34-positive cells are scanty.[32]

Myelodysplastic syndrome associated with an isolated del(5q) chromo-somal abnormality is a distinct entity, predominantly affecting middle-aged or elderly women, which has a more favourable prognosis and prolonged survival.[30] The megakaryocytes are distinctive: they are usually normal or only slightly reduced in size with hypolobated (often monolobated), hyper-chromatic nuclei.

## ACUTE MYELOID LEUKAEMIA

The WHO classification recognises the key role of factors other than morphology in predicting prognosis in haematological malignancies. This is particularly important in acute myeloid leukaemia (AML) in which the presence of specific cytogenetic abnormalities, association with myelo-dysplasia and history of previous cytotoxic chemotherapy all have important prognostic implications. In categorising cases of AML the WHO classification takes a stepwise approach that assesses all of these factors.[33] First, it separates out four disease with recurrent cytogenetic abnormalities associated with a relatively favourable prognosis (Table 4). Next, it separates out those cases in which there is morphological evidence of accompanying multilineage myelodysplasia. Co-existent myelodysplasia is more frequent in older people

**Table 4** The WHO classification of acute myeloid leukaemia (AML)

Acute myeloid leukaemia with recurrent genetic abnormalities
    AML with t(2;21)(q22;q22)
    AML with abnormal bone marrow eosinophils inv(16)(p13q22) or
        t(16;16)(p13;q22)
    Acute promyelocytic leukaemia t(15;17)(q22;q12)
    AML with 11q23 abnormalities
Acute myeloid leukaemia with multilineage dysplasia
Acute myeloid leukaemia and myelodysplastic syndromes, therapy related
Acute myeloid leukaemia not otherwise categorised
    AML minimally differentiated
    AML without maturation
    AML with maturation
    Acute myelomonocytic leukaemia
    Acute monoblastic and monocytic leukaemia
    Acute erythroid leukaemias
    Acute megakaryoblastic leukaemia
    Acute basophilic leukaemia
    Acute panmyelosis with myelofibrosis
    Myeloid sarcoma
Acute leukaemia of ambiguous lineage

and is associated with a poor response to therapy. Disease arising in patients who have a history of cytotoxic chemotherapy, particularly therapy with alkylating agents, are categorised separately. Almost all patients with AML who have had previous alkylating agent therapy have co-existent with myelodysplasia and are refractory to treatment. Finally, patients with AML who do not fall into one of the preceding categories (AML not otherwise categorised) are classified on the basis of the morphology, cytochemistry and immunophenotype of the leukaemic cells on bone marrow aspirate or peripheral blood specimens.[33]

In most cases of AML, bone marrow biopsy histology contributes little extra diagnostic information. In a few cases in which there is marked marrow fibrosis, the bone marrow aspirate is often inadequate and bone marrow trephine biopsy may then play a key role in diagnosis. This is most common in acute megakaryoblastic leukaemia and acute panmyelosis with myelofibrosis.[33] In acute megakaryoblastic leukaemia the bone marrow shows either a diffuse infiltrate of medium-sized blast cells or has blast cells mixed with variable numbers of small dysplastic megakaryocytes. There is usually reticulin fibrosis throughout the stroma. If the fibrosis is severe the appearances can resemble metastatic carcinoma. Immunohistochemical staining for CD42b or CD61 is helpful in confirming the nature of the megakaryoblasts.

Acute panmyelosis with myelofibrosis is a rare subtype of AML in which there is an acute proliferation of all three myeloid cell lines associated with bone marrow fibrosis.[33] There is severe pancytopenia and the clinical course is rapidly progressive. The bone marrow is hypercellular with hyperplasia of all three main haemopoietic cell lineages. Clusters of immature granulocytic precursors including blast cells are often present. Megakaryocytes usually show dysplastic nuclear features. There is a great increase in stromal reticulin. The key feature in distinguishing acute panmyelosis with myelofibrosis from other subtypes of AML is the panmyeloid nature of the proliferation. Rapid clinical evolution, absence of splenomegaly and the presence of small, hypolobated megakaryocytes distinguish acute panmyelosis from chronic idiopathic myelofibrosis.

## MASTOCYTOSIS

The term mastocytosis defines a group of disorders characterised by proliferation of mast cells in one or more organ systems (Table 5).[34,35] There is a wide range of clinical behaviour. At the benign end of the spectrum there are skin lesions that regress spontaneously: at the other end, there are aggressive mast cell neoplasms with systemic, multi-organ involvement. Systemic mastocytosis is defined as disease involving at least one extracutaneous site. Patients in most cases of systemic mastocytosis have bone marrow involvement. Bone marrow infiltration in systemic mastocytosis is characterised by multifocal dense aggregates of mast cells (> 15 cells in each aggregate), confirmed by immunohistochemical staining for mast cell tryptase or c-kit (CD117). More than 25% of the mast cells should be spindle-shaped or have atypical morphology (Fig. 5). Areas of infiltration are usually associated with increased stromal reticulin and, in some cases, collagen fibrosis may be present. There is often an increase in eosinophils and reactive lymphoid cells

**Table 5** The WHO classification of mastocytosis

Cutaneous mastocytosis
Indolent systemic mastocytosis
Systemic mastocytosis with associated clonal haematological non-mast cell
lineage disease
Aggressive systemic mastocytosis
Mast cell leukaemia
Mast cell sarcoma
Extracutaneous mastocytoma

adjacent to the areas of mast cell infiltration. Although cytochemical stains such as toluidine blue and Giemsa will demonstrate cytoplasmic granules in normal and reactive mast cells, these stains may be weak or negative in mastocytosis. We recommend immunohistochemical staining in all trephine biopsies in which the diagnosis is suspected clinically or histologically.

Patients with indolent systemic mastocytosis have a low mast cell burden with less than 30% of bone marrow tissue being replaced and with no evidence of hepatosplenomegaly. Systemic mastocytosis may be associated with clonal haematological malignancy of non-mast cell lineage disease. In such patients, the diagnostic criteria for systemic mastocytosis are met and there is also defining evidence of another clonal disorder (*e.g.* AML, myelodysplasia, chronic myeloproliferative disease or lymphoma). Patients with aggressive systemic mastocytosis have a greater degree of marrow infiltration than indolent systemic mastocytosis with evidence of bone marrow or liver dysfunction or lytic bone lesions. In mast cell leukaemia there is diffuse replacement of normal bone marrow constituents by atypical mast cells accompanied by circulating neoplastic mast cells in the peripheral blood. Mast cell leukaemia has an aggressive clinical course.

## ADVANCES IN LYMPHOPROLIFERATIVE DISORDERS

The new WHO classification incorporates an interesting concept of considering, as part of fundamental disease biology, the recognition that some lymphomas grow

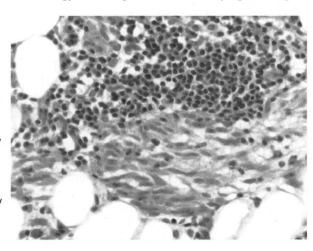

**Fig. 5** Typical bone marrow lesion in indolent mastocytosis. An aggregate of mast cells with atypical spindle cell morphology and hypogranular cytoplasm is present, with a small lymphoid aggregate and eosinophils immediately adjacent. H&E-stained section; original magnification x40.

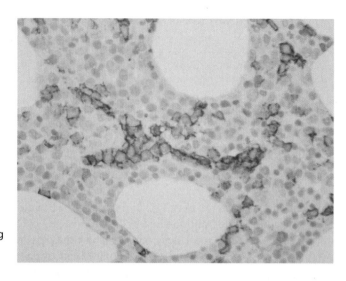

**Fig. 6** Intrasinusoidal infiltration by splenic marginal zone B cell lymphoma. Immuno-histochemical staining for CD20. Original magnification x40.

exclusively or predominantly as solid tumours while others tend to show leukaemic behaviour.[36] The biological basis of this variation is unknown, but abnormal patterns of adhesion molecule expression have been described in several lymphomas and these may contribute. Similarly, the basis of homing patterns of lymphomas to different body tissues remains enigmatic. These aspects of disease behaviour seem likely targets for evolution of the classification in future years. More knowledge of these areas may increase the importance of bone marrow histology in lymphoma diagnosis and prognostication. Currently, the WHO classification mentions a few distinctive bone marrow morphological features associated with particular disease entities (*e.g.* paratrabecular infiltration in follicular lymphoma) but still treats bone marrow trephine biopsy as having essentially a staging function rather than a valuable role in primary diagnosis.

Patterns of bone marrow infiltration by low grade B cell lymphomas have been well described elsewhere.[37] A newly recognised pattern is intrasinusoidal infiltration. This is seen in association with nodular, interstitial or paratrabecular infiltrates in splenic marginal zone lymphoma (Fig. 6).[38–40] As with many new observations, initial optimism that intrasinusoidal infiltration might represent behaviour specific to splenic marginal zone lymphoma or splenic lymphoma with villous lymphocytes (SMZL/SLVL) is probably incorrect. Nonetheless, in the authors' experience, finding this pattern of bone marrow infiltration is strongly associated with a diagnosis of SMZL/SLVL. Other patterns of marrow infiltration by lymphoma can be supportive of rather than specific to the diagnosis of a particular disease. Recognition of intrasinusoidal infiltration is useful even though it is not specific for SMZL/SLVL. Careful attention should always be paid to the morphology and immunophenotype of cells in the sinusoids: intravascular large B-cell lymphoma, a rare subtype of diffuse large B-cell lymphoma, also has this pattern of infiltration in the bone marrow,[41] as does hepatosplenic T-cell lymphoma.

Regrettably, recent advances have not shed much light on the differentiation between reactive lymphoid infiltrates in bone marrow and early involvement by lymphoma or plasma cell neoplasia. Several studies have now used PCR to demonstrate immunoglobulin heavy chain gene clonality in tissue sections from bone marrow containing suspicious bone marrow lymphoid aggregates.[42,43] Successful DNA extraction and PCR amplification have been achieved but false positive and false negative results make this an unreliable technique in this context at present. When one attempts to immunophenotype such aggregates, which are generally small nodules, one may find that further sections prepared for ancillary investigations no longer contain relevant tissue. When such tissue is present, the small number of lymphoid cells may fail to yield a detectable monoclonal product or may permit preferential amplification of a single IgH sequence and so mimic a monoclonal disease. Paratrabecular location of the lymphoid infiltrate within the bone marrow is the most reliable indicator that it is neoplastic. Non-paratrabecular nodules, which are found in most cases, remain a considerable problem. Clinical information and evidence of other reactive features in the marrow, such as interstitial T lymphocytosis, plasmacytosis or increased stromal macrophage activity all require careful consideration subjective opinion about the likely significance of such aggregates can be made.

Better progress is being made in the interpretation of early bone marrow involvement by plasma cell neoplasia.[44] It is still very difficult to interpret plasma cell infiltrates representing 5% or less of nucleated bone marrow cells; these are often found in patients presenting with asymptomatic monoclonal gammopathy.[45] Many such cases are categorised as monoclonal gammopathy of undetermined significance (MGUS) because evidence to confirm neoplasia of plasma cells is lacking. With higher concentrations of plasma cells, neoplastic features have been recognised that correlate with neoplastic behaviour (so-called smouldering myeloma or early multiple myeloma) even in the absence of diffuse bone marrow replacement, intramedullary plasmacytoma formation or bony changes. Clusters of plasma cells replacing all or most of the normal haemopoietic cells between individual adipocytes correlate well with neoplastic plasma cell growth (Fig. 7).[44] Care must be taken to discount plasma cells grouped around stromal capillaries but inter-adipocyte plasma cell clustering is otherwise an extremely helpful indicator of early neoplastic infiltration. The significance of purely pericapillary plasma cell groups is controversial. It is the authors' experience that light chain

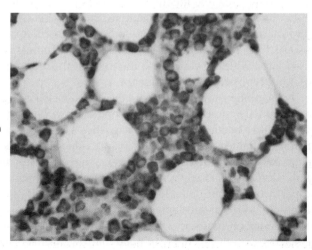

**Fig. 7** Diffuse infiltration of inter-adipocyte tissue in plasma cell myeloma. Immunohistochemical staining for the rough endoplasmic reticulum-associated p63 antigen (antibody VS38c). Original magnification x40.

restriction is rarely, if ever, demonstrable in bone marrow plasma cells showing pericapillary clustering (which may be accompanied by diffusely distributed, singly scattered cells) but no inter-adipocyte clustering. Plasma cell visualisation and quantification in bone marrow trephine sections is greatly aided by immunohistochemical staining for the rough endoplasmic reticulum-associated antigen p63 (antibody VS38c) or for CD138. Kappa and lambda ISH can be performed for confirmation of light chain restriction.

Plasma cell immunophenotype, as well as distribution, may be abnormal in early cases of multiple myeloma. Several flow cytometric studies have indicated that neoplastic plasma cells in some cases of myeloma and MGUS up-regulate expression of CD56, an adhesion molecule (N-CAM) not usually expressed by normal or reactive plasma cells. Highest levels of expression were associated with more aggressive clinical behaviour and greater cytological atypia.[46] The possible usefulness of CD56 immunostaining of plasma cell infiltrates in bone marrow trephine sections has yet to be fully evaluated.

## ADVANCES IN UNDERSTANDING BONE MARROW STROMA

### ORIGIN AND NATURE OF STROMAL CELLS

Experiments performed using bone marrow cell culture have shed considerable light on interactions between stromal and haemopoietic cells in health and disease. Little of this information has so far translated into evidence that can be detected in trephine biopsy sections to assist diagnosis or prognostication. As currently understood, a common mesenchymal precursor cell gives rise to endothelial, fibroblastic and adipogenic marrow stromal cells.[47] This multipotential precursor cell also generates osteoblasts and chondroblasts for bone and cartilage formation. In adult life, stromal cell and haemopoietic cell development is considered, at least in normal marrow, to be from different committed precursor cells. The only normal stromal components to be derived from the multipotential haemopoietic precursors are resident tissue macrophages. However, during embryonic development, a precursor cell can be identified which has the capacity to differentiate along either haemopoietic or angiogenic pathways. This cell, the haemangioblast, is important in morphogenesis of embryonic vasculature as well as in haemopoiesis.[48] It disappears as definitive haemopoiesis moves from structures associated with the yolk sac to the liver; at this time, haemopoietic stem cells of adult type become predominant.

Long-running arguments about the shared or separate origins of haemopoietic and stromal components in adult bone marrow have recently become blurred. Cells with haemangioblast characteristics have been found in patients with chronic granulocytic leukaemia.[49] New evidence about the extreme plasticity of stem cells isolated from several organs suggests that their function is strongly influenced by local environmental controls rather than by irreversible loss of capacity to generate daughter cells of many divergent types. These findings seem likely to lead to development of new therapeutic strategies for stem cell transplantation (with or without manipulation *in vitro*) or induction *in vivo* of desired stem cell functions. In bone marrow, haematopathologists will need to learn to recognise the characteristics and side-effects of haemopoietic reconstitution as a consequence of such interventions.

Our understanding of bone marrow stromal changes in fibrosing diseases such as idiopathic myelofibrosis is still in its early stages. Most marrow fibrosis is reactive, occurring in the context of neoplastic stem cell disease, lympho-proliferative disease or solid tumour metastasis, so it is not surprising that most attention is still focused on the underlying neoplastic process. However, interest in modulating the stromal response to solid tumours elsewhere in the body points the way to considering manipulation of bone marrow stroma for therapeutic effect, particularly in chronic processes such as idiopathic myelofibrosis. In this disease, bone marrow failure due to progressive marrow fibrosis develops in most patients; acute leukaemic transformation occurs in about 15–20%. Factors predictive of bone marrow fibrosis or neo-osteogenesis or both in this context might be very useful in planning clinical management. With the development of wet heat-mediated antigen retrieval techniques, it has become possible to demonstrate non-adipocyte bone marrow stromal cells by their expression of molecules such as CD10 and proteins in the tumour necrosis factor receptor family. The latter include p75 low affinity nerve growth factor receptor (L-NGFR) and the ligand for the receptor activator of nuclear factor kappa-beta (RANK-L).[50,51] A population of cells with dendritic morphology is highlighted, possibly analogous to stellate cells in the liver and pancreas. Whether such stromal cells represent a single, functionally homogeneous population or a mixture is currently unknown. The diagnostic and prognostic potential of detecting changes in number and distribution of these cells is also not yet clear, but is clearly intriguing.

## ANGIOGENESIS IN MARROW STROMA

Interest in angiogenesis associated with solid tumour growth has been considerable in recent years and has led to investigation of bone marrow stromal vascularisation in several haemopoietic cell neoplasms.[52–56] To date, multiple myeloma (MM) has attracted the greatest interest in this area, at least in part because of a desire to explain the effectiveness of thalidomide in the treatment of some patients with this disease. Neovascularisation is seen most extensively infiltrated bone marrow samples in MM.[56,57] The extent of angiogenesis is thought to correlate with progressive disease and to permit distinction between MGUS, early/smouldering myeloma and MM. This has not yet been rigorously tested against other potentially discriminatory criteria in prospective studies. Nevertheless, in active MM, high levels of angiogenesis correlate with a poorer prognosis. Neoplastic plasma cells in MM secrete several angiogenic cytokines, including fibroblast growth factor-2 (FGF-2) and vascular endothelial growth factor (VEGF), which could account for their angiogenic potential.[58] They also secrete increased amounts of matrix metalloproteinase 2 (MMP2) and this might contribute to their invasiveness at intra- and extramedullary sites, as well as to angiogenesis.[58]

Other haemopoietic neoplasms in which increased angiogenesis has been observed include acute lymphoblastic leukaemia (ALL) and B-cell non-Hodgkin's lymphoma.[52,54,55] In ALL, the degree of bone marrow stromal angiogenesis shows no correlation with clinical outcome.[55] The significance of this phenomenon in haematological malignancies is unknown. While acknowledging the success of thalidomide treatment in some patients with MM, its effectiveness has not been formally proven to be due to anti-angiogenic activity.

## BONE MARROW CHANGES WITH NOVEL THERAPIES

Post-therapy changes in bone marrow composition have been studied in many contexts but there has been particular focus in recent years on the effects of defined therapeutic regimens in patients with CML. This emphasis on CML partly reflects practical matters favouring research study. The disease has unambiguous diagnostic criteria and a high frequency of treatment in structured clinical trials. Many such trials require sequential bone marrow trephine biopsy to be performed at specified intervals during treatment. Consequently, excellent data sets may be obtained for histological studies and subsequent clinicopathological correlation. Until very recently, treatment of CML has predominantly involved use of chemotherapeutic agents such as hydroxyurea, given alone or in combination with interferon-α (IFN-α). IFN-α alone has also been used successfully. In CML, IFN-α therapy is associated with progressive fibrosis while hydroxyurea tends to reduce fibrosis.[59–61] Megakaryocytes and their precursors are increased during therapy with IFN-α more than hydroxyurea, associated with development of fibrosis.[60,61] If fibrosis progresses during combined hydroxyurea/IFN-α therapy, this indicates poor outcome and worse survival.[62]

Recent advances in understanding the molecular biology of CML have led to the development of the new tyrosine kinase inhibitor drug STI571 (imatinib mesylate; Glivec). Sequential trephine biopsy in CML patients treated with this agent has shown return to normal megakaryocyte morphology, a normal amount of erythropoiesis and reversal of fibrosis.[63]

Changes in bone marrow of patients with CML treated with allogeneic bone marrow transplantation (aBMT) have also been studied. Higher pre-transplant megakaryocyte and platelet counts in CML correlate with post-transplant reticulin fibrosis and delayed aBMT engraftment.[64,65] Pre-transplant stromal fibrosis in CML regresses transiently post-aBMT but recurs insidiously and is associated with delayed engraftment. Higher levels of early post-transplant fibrosis also correlate with occurrence of severe (grade III/IV) acute graft-versus-host disease.[66]

Experience is limited of the effects of another drug of the molecular biological era, anagrelide. This agent interferes with the interaction between thrombopoietin and its receptor on megakaryocytes, c-mpl. Its use is being evaluated currently for control of platelet production in patients with essential thrombocythaemia. Initial reports suggest that megakaryocyte morphology changes, with loss of large, hypermature forms and an increase of megakaryoblasts and small, immature forms as platelet counts are reduced by this drug.[67]

Use of haemopoietic growth factors for therapy, such as erythropoietin in anaemia due to chronic renal disease, and granulocyte-colony stimulating factor to minimise neutropenia caused by myelosuppressive chemotherapy, has become established in recent years. The contexts of their use are rarely ones in which bone marrow trephine biopsy is indicated. However, G-CSF causes a florid leukaemoid reaction for 2 weeks or more after administration and occasionally catches out unwary haematologists and haematopathologists by close mimicry of CML or CMML.[68,69]

In the history of bone marrow trephine biopsy so far, use of the technique to evaluate changes during and after treatment has been of minor importance. In the last few years, most emphasis has been on expansion of the repertoire of immunohistochemistry and ISH to add value to the histological interpretation of diagnostic bone marrow biopsy specimens. Arrival of the molecular diagnostic era has provided incentives to develop methods to enable use of trephine biopsy tissue as a source of DNA for PCR and there will undoubtedly be further advances in this area for years to come. In addition, increased use of biological response modifiers (cytokines, growth factors and growth factor inhibitors, tyrosine and farnosyl kinase inhibitors) for treatment of haemopoietic diseases in future years will add importance to the role of histology in the assessment of disease progression or responsiveness. There is still new territory for the haematopathologist to discover.

## References

1. Jaffe E, Harris N, Stein H, Vardiman J. (eds). *Pathology and Genetics of Tumours of the Haemopoietic and Lymphoid Tissues. World Health Organization Classification of Tumours.* Lyon: IARC Press, 2001.
2. Frisch B, Bartl R. Biopsy of bone and bone marrow. In: *Biopsy Interpretation of Bone and Bone Marrow; Histology and Immunohistology in Paraffin and Plastic,* 2nd edn. London: Arnold, 1999; 1–11.
3. Wickham C, Boyce M, Joyner M et al. Amplification of PCR products in excess of 600 base pairs using DNA extracted from decalcified, paraffin wax embedded bone marrow trephine biopsies. *J Clin Pathol Mol Pathol* 2000; **53**: 19–23.
4. Sarsfield P, Wickham C, Joyner M et al. Formic acid decalcification of bone marrow trephines degrades DNA: alternative use of EDTA allows amplification and sequencing of relatively long PCR products [Letter]. *J Clin Pathol Mol Pathol* 2000; **53**: 336.
5. Salomen-Nguyen F, Valensi F, Troussard X, Flandrin G. The value of the monoclonal antibody, DBA44, in the diagnosis of B-lymphoid disorders. *Leukoc Res* 1996; **20**: 909–913.
6. Banham A, Turley H, Pulford K, Gatter K, Mason D. The plasma cell associated antigen detectable by antibody VS38 is the p63 rough endoplasmic reticulum protein. *J Pathol* 1997; **50**: 485–489.
7. Mason D, Micklem K, Jones M. Double immunofluorescence labelling of routinely processed paraffin sections. *J Pathol* 2000; **191**: 452–461.
8. Thiele J, Schmitz B, Fuchs R et al. Detection of the *BCR/ABL* gene in bone marrow macrophages in CML and alterations during interferon therapy: a fluorescence *in situ* hybridization study on trephine biopsies. *J Pathol* 1998; **186**: 331–335.
9. Le Maitre C, Byers R, Liu Yin J et al. Dual colour FISH in paraffin wax embedded bone trephines for identification of numerical and structural chromosomal abnormalities in acute myeloid leukaemia and myelodysplasia. *J Clin Pathol* 2001; **54**: 730–733.
10. Lewis F, Maughan N, Smith V et al. Unlocking the archive – gene expression in paraffin-embedded tissue. *J Pathol* 2001; **195**: 66–71.
11. Harris N, Jaffe E, Stein H et al. A revised European-American classification of lymphoid neoplasms: a proposal from the International Lymphoma Study Group. *Blood* 1994; **84**: 1361–1392.
12. Bennett J, Catovsky D, Daniel M et al. Proposals for the classification of the acute leukaemias. French-American-British (FAB) co-operative group. *Br J Haematol* 1976; **33**: 451–458.
13. Bennett J, Catovsky D, Daniel M et al. Proposed revised criteria for the classification of acute myeloid leukemia. A report of the French-American-British Cooperative Group. *Ann Intern Med* 1985; **103**: 620–625.
14. Second MIC Co-operative Study Group. Morphologic, immunologic and cytogenetic (MIC) working classification of the acute myeloid leukaemias. *Br J Haematol* 1988; **68**: 487–494.

15. Bain B, Clark D, Lampert I, Wilkins B. Acute myeloid leukaemia, the myelodysplastic syndromes and histiocytic neoplasms. In: *Bone Marrow Pathology*, 3rd edn. Oxford: Blackwell Science, 2001; 141–190.

16. Bain B, Clark D, Lampert I, Wilkins B. Chronic myeloproliferative and myeloproliferative/myelodysplastic disorders. In: *Bone Marrow Pathology*, 3rd edn. Oxford: Blackwell Science, 2001; 191–230.

17. Vardiman J, Brunning R, Harris N. Chronic myeloproliferative diseases: Introduction. In: Jaffe E, Harris N, Stein H, Vardiman J. (eds). *Pathology and Genetics of Tumours of the Haemopoietic and Lymphoid Tissues. World Health Organization Classification of Tumours.* Lyon: IARC Press, 2001; 17–19.

18. Vardiman J, Pierre R, Thiele J *et al.* Chronic myelogenous leukaemia. Jaffe E, Harris N, Stein H, Vardiman J. (eds). In: *Pathology and Genetics of Tumours of the Haemopoietic and Lymphoid Tissues. World Health Organization Classification of Tumours.* Lyon: IARC Press, 2001; 20–26.

19. Orazi A, Neiman R, Cualing H *et al.* CD34 immunostaining of bone marrow biopsy specimens is a reliable way to classify the phases of chronic myeloid leukemia. *Am J Clin Pathol* 1994; **101**: 426–428.

20. Pierre R, Imbert M, Thiele J *et al.* Polycythaemia vera. In: Jaffe E, Harris N, Stein H, Vardiman J. (eds). *Pathology and Genetics of Tumours of the Haemopoietic and Lymphoid Tissues. World Health Organization Classification of Tumours.* Lyon: IARC Press, 2001; 32–34.

21. Thiele J, Kvasnicka H, Zankovich R, Diehl V. The value of bone marrow histology in differentiating between early stage polycythemia vera and secondary (reactive) polycythemias. *Haematologica* 2001; **86**: 368–374.

22. Thiele J, Pierre R, Imbert M *et al.* Chronic idiopathic myelofibrosis. In: Jaffe E, Harris N, Stein H, Vardiman J. (eds). *Pathology and Genetics of Tumours of the Haemopoietic and Lymphoid Tissues. World Health Organization Classification of Tumours.* Lyon: IARC Press, 2001; 35–38.

23. Thiele J, Kvasnicka H, Boeltken B *et al.* Initial (prefibrotic) stages of idiopathic (primary) myelofibrosis (IMF) – a clinico-pathological study. *Leukemia* 1999; **13**: 1741–1748.

24. Thiele J, Kvasnicka H, Zankovich R, Diehl V. Clinical and morphological criteria for the diagnosis of prefibrotic idiopathic (primary) myelofibrosis. *Ann Hematol* 2001; **80**: 160–165.

25. Imbert M, Pierre R, Thiele J *et al.* Essential thrombocythaemia. In: Jaffe E, Harris N, Stein H, Vardiman J. (eds). *Pathology and Genetics of Tumours of the Haemopoietic and Lymphoid Tissues. World Health Organization Classification of Tumours.* Lyon: IARC Press, 2001; 39–41.

26. Thiele J, Kvasnicka H, Schmitt-Graeff A *et al.*, Follow-up examinations including sequential bone marrow biopsies in essential thrombocythemia (ET): a retrospective clinicopathological study of 120 patients. *Am J Hematol* 2002; **70**: 283–291.

27. Mesa R, Hanson C, Li C *et al.* Diagnostic and prognostic value of bone marrow angiogenesis and megakaryocyte c-MPL expression in essential thrombocythemia. *Blood* 2002; **99**: 4131–4137.

28. Thiele J, Imbert M, Pierre R *et al.* Chronic myeloproliferative disease, unclassifiable. In: Jaffe E, Harris N, Stein H, Vardiman J. (eds). *Pathology and Genetics of Tumours of the Haemopoietic and Lymphoid Tissues. World Health Organization Classification of Tumours.* Lyon: IARC Press, 2001; 42–44.

29. Vardiman J. Myelodysplastic/myeloproliferative diseases: Introduction. In: Jaffe E, Harris N, Stein H, Vardiman J. (eds). *Pathology and Genetics of Tumours of the Haemopoietic and Lymphoid Tissues. World Health Organization Classification of Tumours.* Lyon: IARC Press, 2001; 47–48.

30. Brunning R, Bennett J, Flandrin G *et al.* Myelodysplastic syndromes. In: Jaffe E, Harris N, Stein H, Vardiman J. (eds). *Pathology and Genetics of Tumours of the Haemopoietic and Lymphoid Tissues. World Health Organization Classification of Tumours.* Lyon: IARC Press, 2001; 63–73.

31. Soligo D, Oriani A, Annaloro C *et al.* CD34 immunohistochemistry of bone marrow biopsies: prognostic significance in primary myelodysplastic syndromes. *Am J Hematol* 1994; **46**: 9–17.

32. Orazi A, Albitar M, Heerema N *et al.* Hypoplastic myelodysplastic syndromes can be distinguished from acquired aplastic anemia by CD34 and PCNA immunostaining of bone marrow biopsy specimens. *Am J Clin Pathol* 1997; **107**: 268–274.

33. Brunning R, Matutes E *et al*. Acute myeloid leukaemias.In: Jaffe E, Harris N, Stein H, Vardiman J. (eds). *Pathology and Genetics of Tumours of the Haemopoietic and Lymphoid Tissues. World Health Organization Classification of Tumours*. Lyon: IARC Press, 2001; 76–105.

34. Valent P, Horny H-P, Li CY *et al*. Mastocytosis. In: Jaffe E, Harris N, Stein H, Vardiman J. (eds). *Pathology and Genetics of Tumours of the Haemopoietic and Lymphoid Tissues. World Health Organization Classification of Tumours*. Lyon: IARC Press, 2001; 293–302.

35. Valent P, Horny H-P, Escribano L *et al*. Diagnostic criteria and classification of mastocytosis: a consensus proposal. *Leukoc Res* 2001; **25**: 603–625.

36. Harris N, Jaffe E, Vardiman J *et al*. WHO classification of tumours of hematopoietic and lymphoid tissues: introduction. In: Jaffe E, Harris N, Stein H, Vardiman J. (eds). *Pathology and Genetics of Tumours of the Haemopoietic and Lymphoid Tissues. World Health Organization Classification of Tumours*. Lyon: IARC Press, 2001; 12–13.

37. Bain B, Clark D, Lampert I, Wilkins B. Lymphoproliferative disorders. In: *Bone Marrow Pathology*, 3rd edn. Oxford: Blackwell Science, 2001; 231–331.

38. Franco V, Florena A, Campesi G. Intrasinusoidal bone marrow infiltration: a possible hallmark of splenic lymphoma. *Histopathology* 1996; **29**: 571–575.

39. Labouyrie E, Marit G, Vial J *et al*. Intrasinusoidal bone marrow involvement by splenic lymphoma with villous lymphocytes: a helpful immunohistologic feature. *Mod Pathol* 1997; **10**: 1015–1020.

40. Kent S, Variakojis D, Peterson L. Comparative study of marginal zone lymphoma involving bone marrow. *Am J Clin Pathol* 2002; **117**: 698–708.

41. Gatter K, Warnke R. Intravascular large B-cell lymphoma. In: Jaffe E, Harris N, Stein H, Vardiman J. (eds). *Pathology and Genetics of Tumours of the Haemopoietic and Lymphoid Tissues. World Health Organization Classification of Tumours*. Lyon: IARC Press, 2001; 177–178.

42. Brinckmann R, Kaufmann O, Reinartz B, Dietel M. Specificity of PCR-based clonality analysis of immunoglobulin heavy chain gene rearrangements for the detection of bone marrow involvement by low grade B-cell lymphomas. *J Pathol* 2000; **190**: 55–60.

43. Pittaluga S, Tierens A, Dodoo Y *et al*. How reliable is histologic examination of bone marrow trephine biopsy specimens for the staging of non-Hodgkin lymphoma? A study of hairy cell leukemia and mantle cell lymphoma involvement of the bone marrow trephine specimen by histologic, immunohistochemical and polymerase chain reaction techniques. *Am J Clin Pathol* 1999; **111**: 179–184.

44. Bain B, Clark D, Lampert I, Wilkins B. Multiple myeloma and related disorders. In: *Bone Marrow Pathology*, 3rd edn. Oxford: Blackwell Science, 2001; 332–357.

45. Cesana C, Klersy C, Barbarano L *et al*. Prognostic factors for malignant transformation in monoclonal gammopathy of undetermined significance and smoldering multitype myeloma. *J Clin Oncol* 2002; **20**: 1625–1634.

46. Ely S, Knowles D. Expression of CD56/neural cell adhesion molecule correlates with the presence of lytic bone lesions in multiple myeloma and distinguishes myeloma from monoclonal gammopathy of undetermined significance and lymphoma with plasmacytoid differentiation. *Am J Pathol* 2002; **160**: 1293–1299.

47. Devine S. Mesenchymal stem cells: will they have a role in the clinic? *J Cell Biol* 2002; **38**: 73–79.

48. Choi K. The hemangioblast: a common progenitor of hematopoietic and endothelial cells. *J Hematother Stem Cell Res* 2002; **11**: 91–101.

49. Gunsilius E, Duba H, Petzer A *et al*. Evidence from a leukaemia model for maintenance of vascular endothelium by bone marrow-derived endothelial cells. *Lancet* 2000; **355**: 1688–1691.

50. Wilkins B, Jones D. Immunohistochemical characterisation of intact adherent layers from human long term bone marrow cultures. *Br J Haematol* 1995; **90**; 757–766.

51. Roux S, Meignin V, Quillard J *et al*. RANK (receptor activator of nuclear factor kappa B) and RANKL expression in multiple myeloma. *Br J Haematol* 2002; **117**: 86–92.

52. Ribatti D, Vacca A, De Falco G *et al*. Angiogenesis, angiogenic factor expression and hematological malignancies. *Anticancer Res* 2001; **21**: 4333–4339.

53. Pruneri G, Bertolini F, Soligo D *et al*. Angiogenesis in myelodysplastic syndromes. *Br J Cancer* 1999; **81**: 1398–1401.

54. Kini A, Kay N, Peterson L. Increased bone marrow angiogenesis in B cell chronic lymphocytic leukemia. *Leukemia* 2000; **14**: 1414–1418.

55. Pule M, Gullman C, Dennis D *et al*. Increased angiogenesis in bone marrow of children with acute lymphoblastic leukaemia has no prognostic significance. *Br J Haematol* 2002; **118**: 991–998.

56. Rajkumar S, Mesa R, Fonseca R *et al*. Bone marrow angiogenesis in 400 patients with monoclonal gammopathy of undetermined significance, multiple myeloma and primary amyloidiosis. *Clin Cancer Res* 2002; **8**: 2210–2216.
57. Tricot G. New insights into role of microenvironment in multiple myeloma. *Int J Hematol* 2002; **76 (Suppl 1)**: 334–336.
58. Vacca A, Ribatti D, Roccaro A *et al*. Bone marrow angiogenesis and plasma cell angiogenic and invasive potential in patients with active multiple myeloma. *Acta Haematol* 2001; **106**: 162–169.
59. Thiele J, Kvasnicka H. Comparative effects of interferon and hydroxyurea on bone marrow fibrosis in chronic myelogenous leukemia. *Leukoc Lymphoma* 2001; **42**: 855–862.
60. Thiele J, Kvasnicka H, Schmitt-Graeff A *et al*. Effects of chemotherapy (bisulphan-hydroxyurea) and interferon-alpha on bone marrow morphologic features in chronic myelogenous leukemia. Histochemical and morphometric study on sequential trephine biopsy specimens with special emphasis on dynamic features. *Am J Clin Pathol* 2000; **114**: 57–65.
61. Thiele J, Kvasnicka H, Schmitt-Graeff A *et al*. Effects of interferon and hydroxyurea on bone marrow fibrosis in chronic myelogenous leukemia: a comparative retrospective study multicentre histological and clinical study. *Br J Haematol* 2000; **108**: 64–71.
62. Thiele J, Kvasnicka H, Schmitt-Graeff A *et al*. Therapy-related changes of $CD34^+$ progenitor cells in chronic myeloid leukemia: a morphometric study on sequential trephine biopsies. *J Hematother Stem Cell Res* 2001; **10**: 827–836.
63. Beham-Schmid C, Apfelbeck U, Sill H *et al*. Treatment of chronic myelogenous leukemia with the tyrosine kinase inhibitor STI571 results in marked regression of bone marrow fibrosis. *Blood* 2002; **99**: 381–383.
64. Thiele J, Kvasnicka H, Beelen D *et al*. Megakaryopoiesis and myelofibrosis in chronic myeloid leukemia after allogeneic bone marrow transplantation: an immunohistochemical study of 127 patients. *Mod Pathol* 2001; **14**: 129–138.
65. Thiele J, Kvasnicka H, Beelen D *et al*. Bone marrow engraftment: histopathology of hematopoietic reconstitution following allogeneic transplantation in CML patients. *Histol Histopathol* 2001; **16**: 213–226.
66. Thiele J, Kvasnicka H, Beelen D *et al*. Relevance and dynamics of myelofibrosis regarding hematopoietic reconstruction after allogeneic bone marrow transplantation in chronic myelogenous leukemia: a single center experience on 160 patients. *Bone Marrow Transplant* 2000; **26**: 275–281.
67. Thiele J, Kvasnicka H, Schmitt-Graff A. Anagrelide-induced changes of megakaryopoiesis during therapy of chronic myeloproliferative disorders with thrombocythemia. *Pathologe* 2002; **23**: 426–432.
68. Tegg E, Tuck D, Lowenthal R, Marsden K. The effect of G-CSF on the composition of human bone marrow. *Clin Lab Haematol* 1999; **21**: 265–270.
69. Bain B, Clark D, Lampert I, Wilkins B. Miscellaneous disorders. In: *Bone Marrow Pathology*, 3rd edn. Oxford: Blackwell Science, 2001; 391–429.

## *Further reading*

Bain BJ. Bone marrow aspiration. *J Clin Pathol* 2001; **54**: 657–663.
Bain BJ. Bone marrow trephine biopsy. *J Clin Pathol* 2001; **54**: 737–742.
Bain BJ. Bone marrow biopsy morbidity and mortality. *Br J Haematol* 2003; **121**: 949–51.
Diebold J, Molina T, Camilleri-Broet S, Le Tourneau A, Audouin J. Bone marrow manifestations of infections and systemic diseases observed in bone marrow trephine biopsy review. *Histopathology* 2000; **37**; 199–211.
Lawson S, Aston S, Baker L, Fegan C, Milligan D. Trained nurses can obtain satisfactory bone marrow aspirates and trephine biopsies. *J Clin Pathol* 1999; **52**: 154–156.

*Andrea Buda  Nina Frances Ockendon*
*Massimo Pignatelli*

**11**

# Microsatellite instability and neoplasia

Multiple stages of cellular transformation lead to increased proliferation before a neoplasm is classified as cancer with the possibility of metastasis. A neoplasm is a cell population that has accumulated genetic aberrations which confer selective growth advantages over their non-transformed counterparts, driving dominant clone survival through proliferation and adaptability in the face of an ever-changing environment. Microsatellite instability (MSI) is a characteristic developed by a genome that has undergone modifications which result in an increased rate of mutation accumulation in regions of repetitive DNA sequence. Generally, MSI develops from defects in mammalian mismatch repair (MMR) genes which reduce the capacity of cells to repair specific types of DNA damage. These mutations were first identified in tumours from patients with the familial cancer-predisposition syndrome hereditary non-polyposis colorectal cancer (HNPCC). MSI marks the phenotypic expression of overall elevated mutation rates that can favour survival when growth-controlling genes are mutated.

To understand the concept of MSI, one must first tackle two issues: (i) what is a microsatellite and in what sense is it unstable; and (ii) what mechanisms are modified (activated or inactivated) to cause this instability?

The relation of MSI to generation of neoplastic cell growth can then be traced and hence its relative contribution to the overall process gauged

**Andrea Buda** MD PhD
Post-doctoral Clinical research Fellow, Department of Pathology and Microbiology, Division of Histopathology, University of Bristol, Bristol Royal Infirmary, Malborough Street, Bristol BS2 8HW, UK

**Nina Frances Ockendon** BSc(Hons)
Research Fellow, Department of Pathology and Microbiology, Division of Histopathology, University of Bristol, Bristol Royal Infirmary, Malborough Street, Bristol BS2 8HW, UK

**Professor Massimo Pignatelli** MD PhD FRCPath
Professor of Histopathology, Department of Pathology and Microbiology, Division of Histopathology, University of Bristol, Bristol Royal Infirmary, Malborough Street, Bristol BS2 8HW, UK (for correspondence)

(relative to other contributing factors). The distinction between neoplastic growth and development of cancer should be appreciated though this is often difficult as most relevant understanding of this topic has arisen from the study of tumour tissue that has reached the cancerous state.

It has been argued that defects acting to increase the basal cellular mutation rate are fundamental to tumourigenic progression[1,2] though the notion that a normal mutation rate followed appropriately by clonal expansion would suffice has also been considered.[3] Either way, accelerating the sequential accumulation of genomic defects that constitute full cellular transformation requires an inability to correct genetic code alteration secondary to DNA damage.

## MICROSATELLITE CHARACTERISTICS

### FORM AND STRUCTURAL DISCREPANCIES

It has been found that the coding and the apparently redundant intergenic regions of eukaryotic DNA exhibit stretches of repetitive sequence described as satellite DNA. These usually remain untranscribed and condensed during interphase, constituting the bulk of heterochromatin. Satellite DNA is sub-classified under the terms mini- and microsatellite DNA (see Table 1). This chapter will be concerned predominantly with microsatellite DNA.

Microsatellites are most commonly structured around mono-, di-, or trinucleotide repeats but are known also for tetranucleotides and larger, with the majority of repetitive components being $(CA)_n$. It is known that the human genome contains at least 5000 dinucleotide repeats.[4] A base component repeating twice or more qualifies as one piece of repetitive sequence. The extent of repetition in a microsatellite occurring at a particular locus may remain uniform in every instance (monomorphic) or it may vary greatly in both anthropologic and cellular populations. Such microsatellites are termed polymorphic and can permit distinction between people on the basis of microsatellite size.

Microsatellite function remains largely unknown, especially where occurrence is within intronic DNA. In coding regions, the amino acids encoded are assumed to be necessary for proper functioning of the protein product of the gene. By default of their design, microsatellites can expand and contract in the number of repeats they have by virtue of the intrinsic ease with which

**Table 1** Categories of satellite DNA

| Type of DNA repeat | Number of repeated nucleotides | Total size (bp) |
|---|---|---|
| Satellite | 5–200 | Several million |
| Minisatellite | | |
|     Hypervariable | 10–60 | 1000–20,000 |
|     Telomeric | 6 | 1000–20,000 |
| Microsatellite | 1–4 | < 1000 |

Modified from Bradley J, Johnson D, Rubenstein D. *Molecular Medicine*, 2nd edn. Oxford: Blackwell, 2001.

insertion/deletion frameshifts can occur. Hence, compared with other DNA motifs, they have a tendency to become unstable with respect to their native sequence. Such alterations result mainly from errors in the action of the DNA polymerases following either *de novo* DNA synthesis as part of the replicative process or post-DNA repair of damaged nucleotide regions, but also following recombination. In relation to the accuracy of the polymerase/recombinase, the genetic code plays a fundamental role. Multiple repeats are more difficult to process as they have a tendency to 'slip' when one of the strands 'rides up' over the other causing repeat components to form a loop.[5] Mutation results only if the slipped intermediate is stabilised while the synthetic machinery traverses that stretch of DNA (thus being dependent on the rate of elongation) and if no repair of the error occurs.

## DEVELOPMENT OF MSI

### RELATIVE CONTRIBUTION TO CELLULAR TRANSFORMATION

#### Terms and related conditions

The rapid emergence of knowledge of MSI and related genomic conditions has provided many confusing alternative abbreviations. MSI in humans may also be called MI or MIN. Nucleotide instability (NI or NIN) is the term given to genetic instability induced by defective activity of the nucleotide excision–repair (NER) machinery (see below) which occurs in the skin cancer disease *xeroderma pigmentosum*; it is generated in a similar way to MSI. The difference lies in the mode of DNA damage that is correctable by NER which is mainly exogenously acquired. Chromosomal instability (CI or CIN) describes the situation thought to operate in most human malignancies, in which whole chromosomes may be lost or gained by neoplastic cells through partitioning errors, resulting in aneuploidy.[6] The role of post-mitotic segregation (PMS) genes during genetic division is poorly understood, thus understanding of CI remains in its infancy. CI provides a route to dramatic genetic reorganisation which may be demonstrated by karyotype analysis showing not only alteration of the chromosomal complement but also of the relative association of homologous partners. The cellular 'allelotype' must also be considered. During the development of many neoplasms, loss of heterozygosity (LOH) may occur: one allele of a particular gene is physically lost from individual gene loci or from deletion of larger chromosomal segments. A contribution to carcinogenesis is assumed when there is LOH of one tumour-suppressor gene allele and its counterpart is then inactivated by mutation.

#### Classification of MSI status

Investigation into the degree of MSI found in several tumour tissues has been used to develop specific international criteria for classification of MSI status based on analysis of stability of a panel of five microsatellite markers:[7]

- **Microsatellite stable (MSS)** – the genome does not have instability of its microsatellite DNA and so may have chromosomal instability instead

- **Low microsatellite instability (MSI-L)** – one of five markers shows instability (or < 30–40% of microsatellites if > 5 tested) in which instability is essentially restricted to repeats of two or more nucleotides

- **High microsatellite instability (MSI-H)** – two or more markers are unstable (or $\geq$ 30–40% of microsatellites if > 5 tested). This subtype forms the phenotypic manifestation of a dysfunctional mismatch repair pathway.

### Importance of maintaining genomic stability

Only the primary sequence of the protein-complexed cellular complement of DNA that comprises the human genome will be considered here. The 35,000 or so genes are dispersed throughout the $3 \times 10^9$ base pairs: coding regions (exons) are interlaced with non-coding regions (introns) which themselves must be spliced out to form the functional mRNA from which proteins are translated. The nature of the encryption of amino acids into base triplets is such that the code is degenerate: it allows for 'start', 'stop' and nonsense codons. As this universal encryption is achieved by combination of only four bases in DNA, alteration of one can have dramatic effects on the nature of the protein product, such as the change of an amino acid codon to a stop codon causing premature protein truncation.

The term genomic instability describes not the presence of a mutation state, but an increased tendency to accumulate mutations. It makes no implication of the nature of the alteration or its consequence on cell survival and proliferation. Genomic instability may be contributed to by modification or ablation of any gene which under normal conditions functions to maintain the integrity of the genome.


## DNA DAMAGE AND REPAIR

Causes of disruption of the genetic code include:

- **Environmental (exogenous) agents** – UV light, ionising radiation, genotoxic compounds

- **Metabolic products** – reactive oxygen species, lipid peroxidation wastes

- **Spontaneous degradation of chemical bonds in the DNA ultrastructure** – base deamination or hydrolysis causes miscoding or abasic sites, respectively[8]

- **Replication errors** – DNA loops resulting in insertions, deletions, or base misincorporation by DNA polymerase.

Being continually bombarded by such an array of genomic insults, cells have evolved complex detective (proofreading) and reparative systems to minimise their destructive effects. Mutation, the permanent change of the cell's genetic code, results when the amount of damage accrued by a genome exceeds the capacity for repair that can take place to rectify it.

New pathways of damage detection and repair are continually being discovered, many of which demonstrate collaboration among their component parts.[8]

- **Nucleotide-excision repair (NER) including transcription-coupled repair (TCR) and base-excision repair (BER)** – NER exhibits the widest range of recognition of DNA damage (usually exogenously derived such as by UV radiation) involving global genome NER (GG-NER) or TCR. BER is a related process differing in that it detects predominantly endogenously derived lesions.

- **Homologous recombination and end joining** – these processes repair double-strand breaks such as those caused by ionising radiation and are usually invoked during S and G2, or G1 phases of the cell cycle, respectively.

## MISMATCH REPAIR (MMR)

Identified in prokaryotes many years ago,[9,10] MMR function is crucial to maintaining the clonality of somatic cells, especially those in tissues of high cell turnover such as oesophagogastric and colonic epithelia. MMR operates post-replicatively to correct interbase and insertion/deletion mismatches, including those resulting from slippage of repetitive sequences. In bacteria, MMR comprises three main enzymatic elements – MutS, MutL, and MutH – which act in concert with other enzymes.

- MutS recognises and binds interbase and insertion/deletion mismatches

- MutL associates with MutS and with ATP activates MutH

- MutH is an endonuclease which nicks the error-containing strand providing an insertion point for helicase II (*UvrD*) and single-strand exonucleases; MutH interacts with helicase II to aid loading onto the nick

- Appropriate strand targeting is conferred by the specificity of MutH for unmethylated GATC motifs present in the daughter strand of DNA (immediately post-replication, duplex DNA is hemimethylated)

- Daughter DNA is excised from the GATC as far as the error then re-synthesised by DNA polymerase III holoenzyme, single-strand binding protein, and DNA ligase.

MMR has been conserved throughout evolution, so the fundamentals of the prokaryotic pathway are assumed to form the basis of the eukaryotic system but have greater complexity. Prokaryotic MutS and MutL are homo-oligomeric, whereas the eukaryotic versions function as heterodimers (Fig. 1). The mammalian homologues which have been identified will be considered here.

The mammalian MMR machinery is complemented by five MutS homologues, MSH2–MSH6. The MSH2/MSH6 heterodimer (hMutSα) tends to target 1–2 nucleotide base-base mismatches and 1–10 nucleotide insertion/deletion loops with high affinity, whereas MSH2/MSH3 (hMutSβ) preferentially binds insertion/deletion loops. Thus, they have differing capacities for microsatellite slippage repair, though they both amend +1 and −1 frameshifts.[11] The mammalian MutL homologues identified are MLH1–MLH3, and PMS1 and PMS2 (which are likely to play roles in post-mitotic segregation), and form various heterodimers: MLH1/PMS1 and MLH1/MLH2 have major roles in MMR, and MLH1/MLH3 are apparently of lesser importance. No mammalian equivalent to MutH has yet been identified though the 5′-3′ double-strand exonuclease Exo1 is known to interact with MSH2 and MLH1. Human homologues are denoted by prefix with 'h' (*e.g.* hMLH1).

In addition to the above components, eukaryotic MMR also involves other factors: FEN1; replicating factor C (RFC); replication protein A (RPA), the

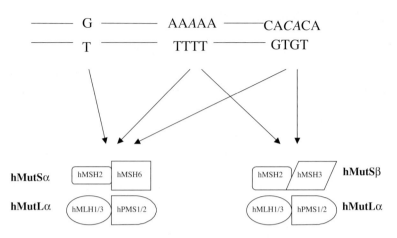

**Fig. 1** Different DNA defects, including base-base mismatches or mono- or dinucleotide insertions (italics), are recognised by alternative combinations of mismatch repair heterodimers. The human homologues functioning in their known capacity are indicated.

eukaryotic equivalent of single-stranded binding protein; proliferating cell nuclear antigen (PCNA); DNA polymerase δ- and ε-associated exonucleases; and DNA polymerase δ. These components do not act exclusively in MMR: they have been implicated in other reparative processes and recombination, acting in conjunction with NER and recombination proteins (Fig. 2).

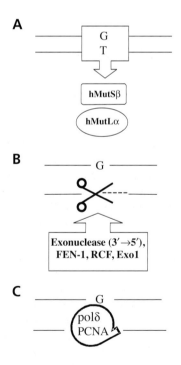

**Fig. 2** Factors involved in the different stages of mismatch repair. (A) Recognition: recruitment of mismatch repair heterodimer to the lesion site. (B) Excision: involving 3′ to 5′ exonuclease action and FEN1, RCF and Exo1 (see text). (C) Re-synthesis: by polymerase δ (polδ) and PCNA.

# MSI RECOGNITION IN NEOPLASIA

## ESTABLISHMENT OF A 'MUTATOR PHENOTYPE'

Many neoplastic cells display genomic instability of one of two forms – chromosomal instability or MSI. Chromosomal instability, resulting in aneuploidy, is the most common accounting for about 85% of colorectal carcinomas. MSI is associated with a near diploid chromosomal constitution. Considering both these conditions, a 'mutator phenotype' of either is thought to operate at some point in most neoplastic progressions. The point at which this progression is initiated is debatable, though the weight of evidence currently favours early transformation.[12] The contribution of chromosomal instability to the initiation of carcinogenesis is readily evident as it provides separate simple events resulting in the loss of numerous alleles, potentially affecting the function of many genes. The underlying contribution of MSI is less apparent: in HNPCC-derived tumours, the germline mutation in the MMR genes accounts for this initial step, but what about in MSI-positive sporadic tumours? Analyses of microsatellite mutations in coding and non-coding regions of sporadic colon cancers by simple sequence repeat PCR have shown tens of thousands of mutations, many of which may be present in the premalignant adenomatous polyp.[13] One study indicated that dysfunction of the MMR genes occurred before mutations of the *APC* gene, a marker for colon cancer, the initiating mutation in the colon cancer predisposing familial adenomatous polyposis (FAP) syndrome.[14]

## SELECTIVE ADVANTAGE OF MSI ON NEOPLASTIC CELL SURVIVAL

The incidence of sporadic neoplasms increases exponentially with age, suggesting the need for 6–12 rate-limiting tumourigenic events[15] to accumulate in one clonal cell population. Each such event would have to confer a selective growth advantage to that population. Considering the oncogenes and tumour suppressor genes now known to be involved in human carcinogenesis, under normal mutation rates only 2 or 3 of these required events would occur. Such occasional incidents cannot be responsible for the development of neoplasms with exorbitant mutation profiles and diverse clonal sub-populations; in these, it is likely that a mutator phenotype has acted. Each transforming stage would provide advantageous features that drive genetic diversification and clonal selection.

Establishment of a mutator phenotype through inactivation of MMR may have its own drawbacks. Just as it may allow initial steps towards transformation, a genome that is unstable reduces the cell's ability to adapt to its environment and may endanger survival. Accumulation of a large number of mutations may be a selective disadvantage and so must be lost if carcinogenesis is to occur.[16] In this way, instability genes (*i.e.* defective MMR genes) are selected for initial growth advantages, then 'hitch-hike' along with such survival factors until the mutations that have been induced threaten cell viability, when they are deselected and lost. A cancer may, therefore, have a confusingly large number of mutations and an apparent absence of MSI: this may be a case of MSI being hidden by deselection.

## HNPCC

HNPCC is the commonest form of hereditary colon cancer, accounting for 5–8% of all colon cancer. It has an autosomal dominant pattern of inheritance and a high penetrance (85–90%), with a life-time risk of colorectal cancer of over 80% (the age of onset is typically < 50 years), which is greater in men. HNPCC may be classified by the site of primary tumour location – type I, exclusively colonic tumours; and type II, extracolonic neoplasms especially in the stomach, endometrium, ovary, and urinary tract.

In 1993, it was shown that people with HNPCC had mutations that mapped to common gene loci.[17] These were later identified as representing components of the MMR machinery, which prompted the definition of a new pathway of colonic carcinogenesis. This was associated with MSI and allows confirmation of diagnosis based on detection of MMR gene mutation. These loci were found to encode the human homologue of the prokaryotic MutS and MutL genes, indicating their important contribution to maintaining the overall stability of the genomic sequence.[17]

That MSI contributes to the progression of sporadic cancers (10–15% of non-familial colorectal cancers have microsatellite instability) has heightened the importance of understanding not only the details of MSI development and its effect on further mutation, but also on its identification. The role of MSI in influencing the final neoplastic phenotype with respect to chemotherapeutic resistance and future metastatic capacity is of importance. Characterisation of a neoplasm according to MMR genotype and MSI status may have a profound influence on the treatment of the tumour.

### Identification of patients at risk for HNPCC: Amsterdam and Bethesda criteria

There is no single clinical feature specific for HNPCC so diagnosis is based on the family history. Criteria were established in 1990 by the International Collaborative Group for HNPCC to establish the clinical diagnosis of HNPCC, referred to as the 'Amsterdam criteria'.[18] These criteria have been criticised for being too strict for clinical application and for not taking into account extracolonic neoplasms that may arise. In response to these comments, the new 'Amsterdam criteria II' were proposed (Box 1).[19]

---

**Box 1 The Amsterdam criteria II**

- three or more family members with an HNPCC-associated cancer (cancer of the ovary, endometrium, stomach, small bowel, liver, bile duct, ureter, or renal pelvis)
- one affected relative as a first-degree relative of two other affected relatives
- cancer extending over two or more generations in the family
- at least one case of familial cancer diagnosed under age 50 years
- pathological verification of all tumours
- being excluded from a familial adenomatous polyposis lineage.

**Box 2  The Bethesda guidelines**

- MSI testing in colorectal tumour specimens is recommended in people with any of the following features:
- cancer in families that meet the Amsterdam criteria
- two HNPCC-related cancers (endometrial, ovarian, gastric, hepatobiliary, small bowel, or transitional cell carcinoma of the renal pelvis or ureter)
- colorectal cancer and a first-degree relative with colorectal cancer and/or HNPCC-related extracolonic cancer and/or colorectal adenoma: one of the cancers diagnosed under 45 years, and the adenoma diagnosed under 40 years
- right-sided colorectal cancer with an undifferentiated pattern (solid-cribiform) on histopathology diagnosed under 45 years
- signet-ring cell type colorectal cancer diagnosed under 45 years
- adenomas diagnosed under 40 years.

The Bethesda criteria consider clinical and histopathological features and have been developed for the identification of MSI in patients with colorectal cancer (Box 2). The Bethesda guidelines permit identification of patients at risk for hereditary cancer and can detect MLH1 and MSH2 germline mutations in patients with colorectal cancer who do not fulfil the Amsterdam criteria.[20]

## LESSONS LEARNED FROM HNPCC – ELUCIDATING THE MECHANISMS OF MMR INACTIVATION LEADING TO MSI

Great efforts have been made to investigate the inactivating events that compromise MMR in neoplasms. Patients presenting with HNPCC usually have heterozygosity for their germline MMR mutations. Biochemical analysis has shown that heterozygosity does not severely affect MMR function and so to develop MSI-H bi-allelic inactivation of at least one of the MMR genes is assumed to be required, in keeping with Knudson's two-hit hypothesis.[21]

Mutations in five different MMR genes have been identified in HNPCC tumours – hMSH2, hMLH1, hPMS1, hPMS2, and hMSH6. Over 90% of cases have hMSH2 or hMLH1 alteration,[22] and are usually classed as MSI-H. The rest includes tumours that have hMSH6 but not hMSH2 or hMLH1 mutations associated with type II HNPCC, with a phenotype characterised by late-onset colorectal cancer presenting with gynaecological tumours, predominantly of the endometrium. These are usually classified as MSI-L tumours. Germline mutation of hPMSI and hPMS2 rarely occur. The characteristics of the most relevant genes and their germline mutations are outlined in Table 2. MSH-H cells tend not to express hMLH1 or hMSH2 protein but most MSI-L and MSS cells have nuclear localisation of these proteins.[22]

**Table 2** Characteristics of MMR genes and their germline mutations

| Gene | Prevalence and classification | Structure | Locus | Mutation features |
|------|------|------|------|------|
| hMSH2 | 40%, MSI-H | 16 exons | 2p22-21 | Mostly unique: single nucleo tide substitutions, deletions or insertions. > 80% cause frame shifts and protein truncations[22] |
| hMLH1 | 40%, MSI-H | 19 exons | 3p21.3 | About 200 mutations identified between exon 15 and 16 cause frameshifts and exon deletion.[23] Single nucleotide substitutions cause splice defects and large genomic deletions.[23] Missense mutations involve the ATPase or the MutL-interacting domain. Those in C-terminal associated with loss of interaction between hMLH1 and hMSH2.[23] All mutations cause unstable transcripts[22] |
| hMSH6 | < 10%, MSI-L | 11 exons | 2p16 | Mutations cluster in the region of hMSH2-interacting domain and the ATP-binding site[23] |

## MSI IN NON-HPCC COLONIC TUMOURS

### MSI-H

In the colon, sporadic MSI-H tumours are prevalent in the proximal colon, occur at a young age, and occur at a higher rate in women. MSI-H cells have several mechanisms of gene de-regulation: (i) germline mutation of 1 allele, LOH/promoter methylation of the remaining allele; (ii) somatic mutation of both alleles; (iii) LOH of 1 allele, promoter methylation of the other; and (iv) bi-allelic methylation (rare).

Most of sporadic MSI-H cancers are caused by silencing of the DNA mismatch repair gene hMLH1. The inactivation of hMLH1 gene in sporadic MSI-H tumours results from methylation of the promoter region and is associated with loss of expression of the hMLH1 protein. A recent study found hypermethylation of the hMLH1 promoter with reduced expression of hMLH1 protein in about 90% of tested MSI-H sporadic cancers.[24]

The morphological features of sporadic MSI-H colonic tumours include a mucinous phenotype of gastric (MUC2) and intestinal (MUC2) mucin in poorly differentiated areas with epithelial cells arranged in irregular clusters. MSI-H seems an independent indicator of good prognosis. Two different studies showed that the 5-year survival rate in patients under 40–50 years of age with MSI-H was significantly higher than with MSS colorectal cancer.[25,26] In one group, the finding was irrespective of tumour stage or grade.[27] The mechanism by which MSI-H could influence the clinical outcome is unknown. A greater severity of MSI might culminate in exceeding an instability threshold, where better prognosis might reflect the final selection pressures incident on such cells: deletion is preferred, perhaps limiting the extent of disease. It is interesting that MSI-H tumours show few mutations of APC, k-ras and p53, genes commonly associated with progression and poor prognosis of colorectal cancer. The intense lymphocytic infiltration observed in MSI-H tumours (including HNPCC) has been associated with the surface expression of non-self antigens. This might result from the accumulation of genetic abnormalities that disrupt normal protein expression and trigger the destruction of cancer cells by the immune system.

Microsatellite instability can also influence the effect of chemotherapeutic agents. *In vitro* studies have shown that MMR-deficient cells are more resistant to many chemotherapeutic drugs, but a recent study has demonstrated that MSI-H is associated with a better sensitivity to 5-fluorouracil and with a better prognosis in patients with stage IV colorectal cancer.[27] The MSI exhibited by cells deficient in hMLH1, hMSH2, and hMSH6 has been shown to be reversibly suppressed by treatment with the non-steroidal anti-inflammatory drugs aspirin and sulindac, the effects being confined to non-apoptotic cells.[28]

## MSI-L

MSI-L and MSS tumours cannot be distinguished morphologically or clinically as they share similar phenotypic and developmental features. They usually have a similar genetic profile, with k-ras and p53 mutations and LOH at 5q, 17p, and 18q frequently detected. Such abnormalities and APC mutations are less common in MSI-H cancers. MSI-L and MSS cells may also present characteristics of the CpG island methylator phenotype (CIMP) but unlike MSI-H cancers, they show methylation of the DNA repair gene $O^6$–methylguanine-DNA methyl transferase (MGMT) in more than 60% of MSI-L cases (discussed below).[29] A particular feature in MSI-L is the association of MGMT methylation with k-ras mutations. It has been suggested that inactivation of MGMT or other MMR genes could result in a mild mutator phenotype predisposing to k-ras mutation.

The proportion of non-MSI-H cancer identified as MSI-L depends on the number of markers used.[30] Recently, MSI analysis using the 13 markers recommended by the Bethesda panel was able to detect only a minority of MSI-L, whereas the use of 44 markers showed MSI-L in nearly 70% of non-MSI-H tumours. This adds weight to the notion that MSI plays a greater role in carcinogenesis that is habitually detected using currently standard techniques. This may be even more extensive as MSI could be being masked by clonal deselection.

## CONTRIBUTION OF METHYLATION

Methylation of DNA CpG islands has been shown to be an important mechanism of gene silencing in some tumour suppressor genes,[31] thus contributing to carcinogenesis. The effect of the genomic methylation status over its ability to maintain microsatellite stability may be considerable, as indicated above for sporadic, late-onset colorectal cancer. It has been suggested that a 'methylator phenotype' may be selected, whereby genes become sensitive to silencing upon methylation of CpG islands in DNA, mostly near the gene promoter.[32] Identification of susceptible regions within the hMLH1 gene promoter and elucidation of the mechanism by which the methylator phenotype contributes to the development of MSI may have important bearings on how the neoplasm progresses and how treatment may be approached.

The MGMT gene, which corrects G–T mismatches after damage by alkylating agents, has been seen to be silenced by methylation, thus allowing lesion persistence.[33] In cells with functional MMR, the extent of repair attempted is futile in the face of the magnitude of the damage and so apoptosis is precipitated (via p53 induction). In MMR-deficient cells, lesion-accumulation remains undetected, apoptosis is avoided, and the clone survives. MGMT silencing seems particularly associated with the MSI-L phenotype.

## TARGET GENES FOR MSI

The markedly higher mutation rate of MSI-H cells, expressed as the 'mutator phenotype' is not necessarily intrinsically transforming. Further mutations to knock out genes that are normally growth suppressing are required to drive transformation. The probability of this occurring in MMR-deficient cells is obviously greater than in MMR-normal cells, hence the relation of MMR function to the initiation and progression of carcinogenesis. This is only so, though, when those genes that are susceptible to mutation via inappropriate repair by MMR are considered (*i.e.* those that contain repetitive sequences).

The first target gene reported for instability in MSI-H colorectal cancer was transforming growth factor β type II receptor (TGFβRII). This gene was shown to be mutated at a poly(A) 10 coding repeat in colonic cancer cell lines and then confirmed in primary MSI-H colorectal cancer.[34] Subsequent studies showed that other genes also have a tendency to develop mutations at repetitive sequences, leading to a new concept of 'target genes' for mutation by microsatellite instability. The observed mutation frequencies in MSI-H tumours reflect the manifestation of the selection pressures on the resultant phenotype. The outcome depends primarily on the function of the gene's protein product but also on the extent of repetition and influence of surrounding sequence, so target genes have been classified according to their contribution to transformation:[35]

- **Survivor genes** – normal function is essential for cell survival genes; therefore, mutations are negatively selected (unless haplo-insufficiency is tolerated)

- **Hibernator genes** – expression is not relevant to the tissue type concerned so phenotypic effects are minimal and selection pressures tend not to act. Mutations in these genes expose the general instability of the condition

- **Co-operator genes** – these cause phenotypic effects only if they synergise with mutations in genes acting in the same pathway; selection is dependent on such additional defects

- **Transformator genes** – mutation provides a *bona fide* step in transformation as a growth advantage is conferred. Positive selection preserves the mutation for clonal expansion, causing mutation frequency to be the highest observed. Examples of such genes include regulators of cell growth (IGFIIR, PTEN) apoptosis (Bax, Fas, Apaf-1), transcription factors (Tcf-4) and components of the Wnt signalling pathway (axin 1, axin 2, Wisp 3).

### MSI and hepatic tumours

Hepatocellular carcinoma is one of the most common malignancies world-wide, where almost all cases develop in the context of cirrhosis or chronic hepatitis. Although risk factors for hepatocellular carcinoma development (hepatitis B [HBV] and C [HCV] infection, cirrhosis of any aetiology, haemocromatosis, and pathological exposure to aflatoxin B) have been well characterised,[35], the subcellular events underlying the complete transformation, in particular the genomic alterations, are not completely understood. Hepatocellular carcinoma has a heterogeneity of genomic lesions, probably contributed to by genetic and epigenetic incidents disrupting many regulatory pathways.[37]

MSI has been identified in hepatocytes of chronic hepatitis, cirrhosis and hepatocellular carcinoma: mutated microsatellite loci have been identified in cirrhotic and dysplastic nodules, and in adjacent hepatocellular carcinoma, supporting the notion that the carcinoma arises from a monoclonal population of dysplastic hepatocytes with a specific genetic alteration.[38] Protein products of HBV and HCV genes are thought to impair the function of enzymes involved in DNA repair leading to failure to correct insertion/deletion mismatches and other frameshift mutations which can result in a cell population with an increased mutation rate.

### MSI in gynaecological tumours

Endometrial and colorectal cancers have many phenotypic similarities. Several lines of evidence suggest that endometrial cancer develops through the hyperplasia-adenoma-carcinoma pathway as a consequence of the accumulation of genetic changes involving tumour suppressor genes such as k-ras and p53.[39] Indeed, endometrial cancer occurs frequently in patients with HNPCC. The incidence of MSI in endometrial cancer varies from 17–32% of sporadic tumours to more than 75% when associated with HNPCC.[40,41] The tumour suppressor gene PTEN, which induces cell cycle arrest and promotes apoptosis, has been implicated in human carcinogenesis; it is unstable at a particular microsatellite locus. PTEN is mutated in more than 80% of cases of endometrial cancer, particularly in the endometrioid subtype.[42] Mutations in PTEN have been also detected in normal-appearing endometrium exposed to oestrogen and in 18–55% of pre-cancerous endometrial lesions.[43]

### MSI in bladder cancer

Bladder carcinoma is the most common urothelial malignancy and is characterised by a high recurrence rate ranging from 50–80% in the 2 years after tumour resection.[44] The occurrence of MSI and MMR deficiencies in bladder cancer have been reported.[45,46] Allelic loss in hMLH1 and hMSH2 and abnormalities in the expression of their protein products (detected by immunohistochemical analysis) have been demonstrated in transitional and squamous cell bladder cancers. In most cases, a reduced expression rather than absence of hMLH1 and hMSH2 was found, suggesting, as for other sporadic cancer, that the deficiency of the MMR system could be a late event in tumour progression.[47]

Earlier studies demonstrated the value of microsatellite analysis in detecting bladder cancer. A non-invasive molecular diagnostic method testing exfoliated cells in urine has been shown to be highly sensitive in detecting primary tumours and recurrences.[48]

## IDENTIFICATION OF MSI

### MSI ANALYSIS

MMR deficiency has been observed in many cases of sporadic cancers as well as hereditary syndromes, so determination of MSI status is an efficient approach for detecting malignancies. The MSI status can then help to place the tumour origin in the context of how the transformation-initiating mutations came to occur. International criteria for diagnosis of MSI have been developed by the National Cancer Institute. They recommend analysis of at least 5 different markers including two mononucleotide repeats (BAT 25 and BAT 26) and three dinucleotide repeats (D2S123, D5S356 and D17S250). More reliable results can be obtained using DNA from fresh tissue, but testing can also be done on DNA from paraffin-wax embedded, formalin-fixed tissue. Normal DNA and tumour DNA from the same patient are needed and constitutional DNA from family members should be examined for germline mutation analysis of the relevant MMR genes.

MSI can be detected by PCR amplification of microsatellite loci in DNA extracted from a variety of pathological material. To improve accuracy and reproducibility of MSI analysis, a new technique using nucleic acid fluorescence labelling and laser scanning has been introduced. Recently, fluorescence PCR amplification has also been applied successfully for MSI analysis using haematoxylin-eosin-stained tissue.

### IMMUNOHISTOCHEMISTRY

A growing body of evidence indicates that immunohistochemical detection of hMLH1 and hMSH2 protein products using commercially available monoclonal antibodies is a straightforward, sensitive and specific technique. IHC in combination with MSI testing has proved to be an extremely useful tool that can dramatically improve the clinical interpretation of germline results. Loss of expression of either hMSH2 and hMLH1 proteins correlates highly with MSI-H: immunohistochemical analysis provides important diagnostic information and could specify which of the two genes is most likely mutated. Loss of expression of MMR protein has been detected by immunohistochemistry in adenomas of HNPCC patients with low levels of MSI.

### MMR GENE TESTING

Delving deeper than the reaches of IHC and MSI testing, direct gene analysis can illustrate the precise inactivation event that has occurred. Several methods are used as specific defects are detected with varying efficiency according to the methodology employed. These may include: (i) protein truncation testing; (ii) single-stranded conformational polymorphism; (iii) denaturing gradient gel electrophoresis; (iv) reverse transcriptase-PCR; (v) conformation sensitive gel electrophoresis; and (vi) direct gene sequencing.

The sensitivity of protein truncation testing for MMR gene mutations is low; therefore, direct sequencing, conformation sensitive gel electrophoresis or single-stranded conformational polymorphism are recommended instead.

## Points for best practice

- MSI is a genomic defect in which microsatellite loci undergo increased mutation rates – the number of repeats expands or contracts. This is due to reduced function of the MMR genes, mostly the hMSH2 and hMLH1.

- MMR gene inactivation may be through genetic or epigenetic mutations – the primary gene sequence is altered so the protein is not expressed (or is in a mutant form), or gene expression is silenced through promoter methylation.

- MSI is associated with a diploid or near diploid karyotype unlike chromosomal instability, in which loss of heterozygosity occurs resulting in aneuploidy.

- Characterisation of MSI status by DNA analysis can help in understanding tumour origin, distinguishing primary from metastasised tumour tissue, and predicting outcome in certain cancers (e.g. colorectal cancer).

- Immunohistochemistry in combination with MSI testing improves the clinical relevance of germline results from DNA analysis.

### References

1. Loeb LA. Mutator phenotype may be required for multistage carcinogenesis. *Cancer Res* 1991; **51**: 3075–3079.
2. Hartwell L. Defects in a cell cycle checkpoint may be responsible for the genomic instability of cancer cells. *Cell* 1992; **71**: 543–6.
3. Tomlinson IP, Novelli MR, Bodmer WF. The mutation rate and cancer. *Proc Natl Acad Sci USA* 1996; **93**: 14800–14803.
4. Kunzler P, Matsuo K, Schaffner W. Pathological, physiological, and evolutionary aspects of short unstable DNA repeats in the human genome. *Biol Chem* 1995; **376**: 201–211.
5. Streisinger G, Okada Y, Emrich J et al. Frameshift mutations and the genetic code. *Cold Spring Harb Symp Quant Biol* 1966; **31**: 77–84.
6. Mitelman F, Johansson B, Mertens F. *Catalog of Chromosome Aberrations in Cancer*, vol. 2. New York: Wiley-Liss, 1994.
7. Boland CR, Thibodeau SN, Hamilton SR et al. A National Cancer Institute Workshop on Microsatellite Instability for cancer detection and familial predisposition: development of international criteria for the determination of microsatellite instability in colorectal cancer. *Cancer Res* 1998; **58**: 5248–5257.
8. Hoeijmakers JHJ. Genome maintenance mechanisms for preventing cancer. *Nature* 2001; **411**: 366–374.
9. Friedberg EC, Walker GC, Siede W. *DNA Repair and Mutagenesis*. Washington, DC: ASM Press; 1995.
10. Modrich P. Mechanisms and biological effects of mismatch repair. *Annu Rev Genet* 1991; **25**: 229–253.
11. Harfe BD, Jinks-Robertson S. DNA mismatch repair and genetic instability. *Annu Rev Genet* 2000; **34**: 359–399.
12. Loeb LA. A mutator phenotype in cancer. *Cancer Res* 2001; **61**: 3230–3239.
13. Stoler DL, Chen N, Basik M et al. The onset and extent of genomic instability in sporadic colorectal tumor progression. *Proc Natl Acad Sci USA* 1999; **96**: 15121–15126.
14. Huang J, Papadopoulos N, McKinley AJ et al. APC mutations in colorectal tumors with mismatch repair deficiency. *Proc Natl Acad Sci USA* 1996; **93**: 9049–9054.

15. Armitage P, Doll R. The age distribution of cancer and a multistage theory of carcinogenesis. *Br J Cancer* 1954; **8**: 1–12.

16. Eigen M. The origin of genetic information: viruses as models. *Gene* 1993; **135**: 37–47.

17. Fishel R, Lescoe MK, Rao MR *et al*. The human mutator gene homolog MSH2 and its association with hereditary nonpolyposis colon cancer. *Cell* 1993; **75**: 1027–1038.

18. Vasen HF, Mecklin JP, Khan PM, Lynch HT. The International Collaborative Group on Hereditary Non-Polyposis Colorectal Cancer (ICG-HNPCC). *Dis Colon Rectum* 1991; **34**: 424–425.

19. Vasen HF, Watson P, Mecklin JP, Lynch HT. New clinical criteria for hereditary nonpolyposis colorectal cancer (HNPCC, Lynch syndrome) proposed by the International Collaborative Group on HNPCC. *Gastroenterology* 1999; **116**: 1453–1456.

20. Rodriguez-Bigas MA, Boland CR, Hamilton SR *et al*. A National Cancer Institute Workshop on Hereditary Nonpolyposis Colorectal Cancer Syndrome: meeting highlights and Bethesda guidelines. *J Natl Cancer Inst* 1997; **89**: 1758–1762.

21. Knudson Jr AG. Mutation and cancer: statistical study of retinoblastoma. *Proc Natl Acad Sci USA* 1971; **68**: 820–823.

22. Yuen ST, Chan TL, Ho JW *et al*. Leung germline, somatic and epigenetic events underlying mismatch repair deficiency in colorectal and HNPCC-related cancers. *Oncogene* 2002; **21**: 7585–7592.

23. Jacob S, Praz F. DNA mismatch repair defects: role in colorectal carcinogenesis. *Biochimie* 2002; **84**: 27–47.

24. Miyakura Y, Sugano K, Konishi F *et al*. Extensive methylation of hMLH1 promoter region predominates in proximal colon cancer with microsatellite instability. *Gastroenterology* 2001; **121**: 1300–1309.

25. Lukish JR, Muro K, DeNobile J *et al*. Prognostic significance of DNA replication errors in young patients with colorectal cancer. *Ann Surg* 1998; **227**: 51–56.

26. Gryfe R, Kim H, Hsieh ET *et al*. Tumor microsatellite instability and clinical outcome in young patients with colorectal cancer. *N Engl J Med* 2000; **342**: 69–77.

27. Liang JT, Huang KC, Lai HS *et al*. High-frequency microsatellite instability predicts better chemosensitivity to high-dose 5-fluorouracil plus leucovorin chemotherapy for stage IV sporadic colorectal cancer after palliative bowel resection. *Int J Cancer* 2002; **101**: 519–525.

28. Ruschoff J, Wallinger S, Dietmaier W *et al*. Aspirin suppresses the mutator phenotype associated with hereditary nonpolyposis colorectal cancer by genetic selection. *Proc Natl Acad Sci USA* 1998; **95**: 11301–11306.

29. Whitehall VL, Walsh MD, Young J, Leggett BA, Jass JR. Methylation of O-6-methylguanine DNA methyltransferase characterizes a subset of colorectal cancer with low-level DNA microsatellite instability. *Cancer Res* 2001; **61**: 827–830.

30. Jass JR, Whitehall VL, Young J, Leggett BA. Emerging concepts in colorectal neoplasia. *Gastroenterology* 2002; **123**: 862–876.

31. Gonzalgo ML, Jones PA. Mutagenic and epigenetic effects of DNA methylation. *Mutat Res* 1997; **386**: 107–118.

32. Toyota M, Ahuja N, Ohe-Toyota M *et al*. CpG island methylator phenotype in colorectal cancer. *Proc Natl Acad Sci USA* 1999; **96**: 8681–8686.

33. Esteller M, Hamilton SR, Burger PC, Baylin SB, Herman JG. Inactivation of the DNA repair gene O6-methylguanine-DNA methyltransferase by promoter hypermethylation is a common event in primary human neoplasia. *Cancer Res* 1999; **59**: 793–797.

34. Markowitz S, Wang J, Myeroff L *et al*. Inactivation of the type II TGF-beta receptor in colon cancer cells with microsatellite instability. *Science* 1995; **268**: 1336–1338.

35. Duval A, Hamelin R. Mutations at coding repeat sequences in mismatch repair-deficient human cancers: toward a new concept of target genes for instability. *Cancer Res* 2002; **62**: 2447–2454.

36. Thorgeirsson SS, Grisham JW. Molecular pathogenesis of human hepatocellular carcinoma. *Nat Genet* 2002; **31**: 339–346.

37. Macdonald GA, Greenson JK, Saito K, Cherian SP, Appelman HD, Boland CR. Microsatellite instability and loss of heterozygosity at DNA mismatch repair gene loci occurs during hepatic carcinogenesis. *Hepatology* 1998; **28**: 90–97.

38. Kondo Y, Kanai Y, Sakamoto M, Mizokami M, Ueda R, Hirohashi S. Genetic instability

and aberrant DNA methylation in chronic hepatitis and cirrhosis – A comprehensive study of loss of heterozygosity and microsatellite instability at 39 loci and DNA hypermethylation on 8 CpG islands in microdissected specimens from patients with hepatocellular carcinoma. *Hepatology* 2000; **32**: 970–979.

39. Ichikawa Y, Lemon SJ, Wang S, Franklin B, Watson P, Knezetic JA *et al.* Microsatellite instability and expression of MLH1 and MSH2 in normal and malignant endometrial and ovarian epithelium in hereditary nonpolyposis colorectal cancer family members. *Cancer Genet Cytogenet* 1999; **112**: 2–8.

40. Risinger JI, Berchuck A, Kohler MF, Watson P, Lynch HT, Boyd J. Genetic instability of microsatellites in endometrial carcinoma. Cancer Res 1993; **53**: 5100–3.

41. Burks RT, Kessis TD, Cho KR, Hedrick L. Microsatellite instability in endometrial carcinoma. *Oncogene* 1994; **9**: 1163–1166.

42. Zhou XP, Kuismanen S, Nystrom-Lahti M, Peltomaki P, Eng C. Distinct PTEN mutational spectra in hereditary non-polyposis colon cancer syndrome-related endometrial carcinomas compared to sporadic microsatellite unstable tumors. *Hum Mol Genet* 2002; **11**: 445–450.

43. Mutter GL, Lin MC, Fitzgerald JT *et al.* Altered PTEN expression as a diagnostic marker for the earliest endometrial precancers. *J Natl Cancer Inst* 2000; **92**: 924–930.

44. Stein JP, Grossfeld GD, Ginsberg DA *et al.* Prognostic markers in bladder cancer: a contemporary review of the literature. *J Urol* 1998; **160**: 645–659.

45. Mao L, Schoenberg MP, Scicchitano M *et al.* Molecular detection of primary bladder cancer by microsatellite analysis. *Science* 1996; **271**: 659–662.

46. Gonzalez-Zulueta M, Ruppert JM, Tokino K *et al.* Microsatellite instability in bladder cancer. *Cancer Res* 1993; **53**: 5620–5623.

47. Kassem HS, Varley JM, Hamam SM, Margison GP. Immunohistochemical analysis of expression and allelotype of mismatch repair genes (hMLH1 and hMSH2) in bladder cancer. *Br J Cancer* 2001; **84**: 321–328.

48. Steiner G, Schoenberg MP, Linn JF, Mao L, Sidransky D. Detection of bladder cancer recurrence by microsatellite analysis of urine. *Nat Med* 1997; **3**: 621–624.

# Index